SOPHIE'S STORY

My 20-Year Battle with Irritable Bowel Syndrome

SOPHIE LEE

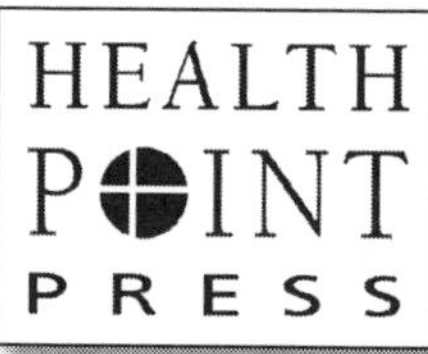

The information and advice contained in this book are based upon the research and the personal experiences of the author. They are not intended as a substitute for consulting with a health care professional. The publisher and author are not responsible for any adverse effects or consequences resulting from the use of any of the suggestions, preparations, or procedures discussed in this book. All matters pertaining to your physical health should be supervised by a health care professional. It is a sign of wisdom, not cowardice, to seek a second or third opinion.

EDITOR: Kathleen Barnes
COPYEDITOR: Lisa Kaspin
COVER, INTERIOR FORMATTING & DESIGN: Gary A. Rosenberg

Health Point Press
4335 Van Nuys Blvd
Sherman Oaks, CA 91403
818-788-2040 • www.healthpointpress.com

The Library of Congress Cataloging-in-Publication data is available through the Library of Congress.

ISBN: 978-0-9826183-2-5

Printed in the United States of America

10 9 8 7 6 5 4 3 2 1

Contents

To my mum and dad

Acknowledgments

This book is dedicated to my wonderful, loving, sweet and supportive mum and dad. You have watched over me through years of illness, and I would never have made it without you.

A big thank you to my publisher, David Knight. I am so thankful to have found a publisher who has such a genuine understanding of IBS.

And a heartfelt thank you to every single IBS sufferer who has contacted me since I launched the IBS Tales website. Discovering that my painful and embarrassing symptoms were shared by so many thousands of other people was a great relief. Discovering that so many of my fellow sufferers are kind, generous and thoughtful was even better.

Introduction

I'VE HAD IRRITABLE BOWEL SYNDROME FOR TWENTY YEARS. For most of my life I have lived with urgent diarrhea, horrible constipation and agonizing stomach pain. I have spent whole afternoons in the bathroom, and on my very worst days I have endured vicious attacks that left me shaking, sweating and scared.

I have regularly broken down in tears because my symptoms were so unforgiving and so constant. I have lost friends because I had no way to explain why I was so reluctant to go on holiday or eat certain foods or plan things in advance. At one point I nearly lost my entire career. I've been told that my symptoms are all in my head and that I should ignore them and get on with my life. While I saw IBS as a nightmare, my doctors saw it as a minor inconvenience.

And I'm not alone. Millions of other IBS sufferers all over the world share my experiences.

This book chronicles my long battle with IBS. It gives me the chance to explain that IBS is a difficult, embarrassing and painful experience. If you or someone you love is a fellow sufferer, I'm so sorry you have to deal with this too.

When the world tells us that IBS is a psychological disorder or that we just need to relax and stop worrying, we need to fight back. This book is my way of fighting back.

I want to tell the absolute truth about IBS, because the reality of this disorder is so often clouded by embarrassment and myths. Perhaps the most pervasive myth is that IBS means mild diarrhea and nothing more. Many people with no experience of IBS wonder why we have such difficulty in coping with our condition. This book shows why.

I'm not ashamed to tell the truth, not remotely, not anymore. IBS has been such a big part of my life that my gravestone will probably read, "Here lies Sophie Lee, who spent most of her time in the bathroom," but I've had as much control over IBS as I have over the fact that I need glasses. I refuse to be embarrassed by a problem that is not of my making.

In addition, I want to offer hope. Although it has taken me many years, I have finally found relief from IBS. IBS patients may well suffer for years, but we still carry on with our lives and make it through. Along the way, many of us find ways to beat our symptoms and take back control of our lives. The amount of strength this requires is very rarely recognized.

So if you're struggling with pain or marathon bathroom sessions or awful constipation, I would like you to know that I admire you a great deal just for living your life with the IBS monster. One day, I hope you kill the beast.

Disclaimer

This book has been written entirely by me. I have had IBS for many years, and this book is a record of my personal experiences and thoughts on IBS. However, this book does *not* offer any medical advice and should not be used to diagnose or treat any medical condition. I accept no responsibility if you try a treatment mentioned in this book and then drop down dead or metamorphose into any kind of fruit bat. If you are experiencing any bowel symptoms, please see a doctor.

CHAPTER 1

A Difficult Beginning for a 12-Year-Old

I WAS 12 WHEN IT ALL BEGAN. One night I developed the worst stomachache that I had ever experienced in my life, with a pain so intense it kept me awake until the early hours of the morning. I didn't get up and tell my parents that I was ill because I thought that the pain would be gone by the morning, and eventually I managed to drop off to sleep.

A few hours later I woke up to find myself vomiting all over the bedclothes and down the side of the bed. It was a suitably dramatic beginning to the single most influential event of my life.

I got out of bed to go vomit some more in the bathroom, and my parents must have heard the noise because they came and helped me clean myself up and get back to bed. I remember feeling relieved that I had gotten through the worst of it, thrown up the last of it, and would now be able to sleep.

The purging seemed to calm my stomach, and I managed to go back to sleep. However, when I woke up in the morning, things were much worse. Although my stomach felt fine, I was actually so ill that I barely realized I had suffered from diarrhea during the night and stained the bedclothes. When I went to see my parents to tell them I was feeling much better, I immediately had to run back to the toilet and vomit again.

The whole of the next day I had to lie on a trash bag to prevent my incontinence from staining the bedsheet. Throughout the day, I alternately vomited into a dishpan and soiled myself with uncontrollable diarrhea.

I am sure you are enjoying reading this as much as I enjoyed participating in it. And I am sure my poor mum, who had to clean up after me, enjoyed it even more. Thanks, Mum.

After a few more cycles of vomiting and diarrhea, I eventually felt better, recovered my strength over a weekend and went back to school on Monday feeling grateful that the whole nasty experience was behind me. Little did I know that those few days had probably sown the seed for years of gut trouble.

I never found out what caused this dramatic bout of sickness, but it seems likely that it was food poisoning, although no one else in my family became ill. I'm not sure why my parents didn't call the doctor, but I guess it was because they knew that the doctor was going to tell them to keep doing what they were doing already: look after me, make me rest and wait for it to pass.

The one positive thing I can say is that this event gave me a definitive starting point for my symptoms, and a classic one at that. Many IBS sufferers date their symptoms back to a food-poisoning incident or major stomach upset.

Knowing what started your IBS doesn't mean that your symptoms will be more easily treated. However, it is at least a little reassuring to know that my symptoms had a logical beginning, and the years of suffering that followed were a kind of post-traumatic bowel syndrome, if you will, or a perfectly normal long-term reaction to a very extreme event.

Although the food-poisoning incident was the true starting point for my symptoms, the IBS started attacking me quietly, insidiously, rather than mounting an all-out assault. When I returned to school, I felt fine, and that was how I felt for most of the time. But something subtle had shifted inside of me, and I began to feel its effects.

Before we go any further, I should probably tell you a little bit about my background. Some doctors believe that all IBS patients come from broken and abusive homes, because that would allegedly explain why we grow up to be so anxious about our bowels (never mind that we are so anxious about our bowels because they're so broken), so I'd like to stake my claim to having possibly the most normal childhood in the history of the world.

I grew up in the county of Hampshire on the south coast of England. We moved to Hampshire when I was about three years old, and I can't remember living anywhere else.

I have a mother and father (who are married, if you're interested, and not to other people) and one older brother. We lived in a four-bedroom house in a nice suburb of a nice town. We went on holiday to France and Wales and Devon, played together in the garden and ate together at mealtimes. My parents were loving and sweet and always came to parents' evenings and music recitals. My dad liked old cars and my mum liked knitting. My dad once bought me a three-foot-tall teddy bear during his lunch hour and carried it back to his office while wearing his best business suit. (I got the bear for Christmas and called him Barney.) I once drew my mum a picture that showed her trademark red hair and the words underneath, "I love my mummy and she loves me."

I liked music, books, my hamster Horace, my tortoise Jason, the family cat Curry (who I wanted to call Biscuit, a superior name), telly and macaroni cheese with bacon. I was very happy at school and got good grades. One school report said, "You work so very quietly, Sophie—we hardly know you're there!" and I never, ever got into trouble.

I should, by all accounts, be the best-adjusted person in the universe. (If there are any psychiatrists reading this who are thinking, *Ah yes, you clearly had such a normal childhood that it went right round the other side and came out damaging,* then all I have to say is, "Sorry guys, but you can't have it both ways.")

I was a happy child and I took my health completely for granted. I don't remember having any problems with my stomach before the food-poisoning incident or ever having diarrhea or constipation. I would occasionally get ill, but I would soon recover and be none the worse for wear. I lived a perfectly healthy, normal life—and then things changed.

Over the next few months I started to suffer from frequent stomachaches and cramps. Perhaps the first major episode occurred one night at a friend's sleepover party, when I couldn't believe how much my stomach hurt. At the time I innocently thought that it could have had something to do with the fact that I'd spent the evening being jumped on and hit with a pillow (we were 12). There's no doubt in my mind now that it was a standard-issue IBS pain attack, albeit without any accompanying diarrhea or constipation.

As well as this first ever episode of pain, I started to experience day-to-day digestive symptoms that were very draining. I began to notice a correlation between how my stomach felt and how recently I had been to the bathroom. I had never suffered from constipation before, but I soon realized that whenever I missed a day's bowel movement, I would feel very tight around my stomach and generally feel ill.

I was far too embarrassed to tell anyone about my newly developed problems and I kept them very much to myself. I did pluck up the courage to buy some over-the-counter laxatives, which helped a little, although they also made my stomach hurt and tended to cause major diarrhea rather than a normally functioning bowel.

I don't really know what I thought was happening to me, or why I was feeling so ill. I had never heard of IBS, and I had never spoken to an IBS sufferer in my life. Even the idea that my symptoms might indicate something more than random stomach upsets didn't really occur to me. I guess I just accepted that I now had a less-than-impressive digestive tract and was going to have to get used to it.

I certainly wasn't worried about having something like bowel cancer or a "serious" illness; I really have no idea why. It should go without saying, of course, but anyone who has symptoms like this and doesn't see a doctor is being a bit loony tunes. In my defense, I was very young and rather mortified, so keeping quiet seemed to be the only option available.

My newly acquired gut problems began to affect every aspect of my life and started to ruin experiences that should have been fantastic. One of the most memorable was a school trip where we were taken to the south of France. It was an activity holiday, canoeing and surfing and all things like that, which wasn't really my scene, but I wanted to go because my friends were going. I was 14 by this stage.

My biggest problem on this holiday involved the toilets. The campsite where we were staying only had open-plan, public toilet-type bathrooms, which meant that if you wanted to have a bowel movement you had to do it with twelve other people standing outside talking, waiting for you to finish and filming you with a camcorder (well, not that last bit, but you get the general idea).

For an IBS person this is the seventh circle of hell, for a number of reasons. Firstly, you never know if you are going to need two minutes or two hours in the bathroom to be finished. Secondly, your body might come up with all kinds of interesting smells to accompany your time in the cubicle, and thirdly, there's a good chance that an IBS bowel will at any time produce a sound only slightly less alarming than a foghorn. Crapping successfully was really quite out of the question.

So I did what any self-respecting constipated person would do: I didn't go to the bathroom for four days. By the end of that time, I felt terrible.

This would be the first of many, many holidays and trips that would be spoiled by my IBS. Many perfectly healthy people find that their bowels shut down on holiday or when their routine has changed and others find that their bowels go crazy and they can't leave the hotel. If you have IBS, these travel-related symptoms can be multiplied a hundredfold, leaving your bowel in a terrible state.

On the fifth day of the holiday, we were packing up to go to another campsite when I finally went to the toilet. I still had another week of holiday to survive. I remember sitting on some steps, looking at my classmates joking and laughing around me, thinking, *Why the hell do I have to deal with this when you lot are so carefree? What have I ever done to deserve it?*

In the end, things were a bit better for me at the second campsite. There were still communal toilets, but my bowel decided to give me a break and actually worked fairly normally for once. So I made it through that experience, but with far more stress and pain than a 14-year-old on holiday really deserves, I think.

Another ruined holiday was with a friend of mine from school and her family and again we went to France. We drove to Dover in the evening and got the overnight ferry. I was in trouble with my stomach before we had even reached France. I remember sitting alone in the bathroom at midnight thinking how much easier life would be if I could just have a working bowel.

The next day we spent hours traveling in the car, stopping at a bed and breakfast in the evening. That night I decided to take some laxative pills, because it looked like I might never go to the bathroom again and therefore explode, and that seemed a sequence of events best avoided. Making sure that my friend didn't see me, I swallowed the pills. Luckily for me they worked while we were still at the bed and breakfast rather than when we were in the car, and it was doubly lucky that the bathroom was on the floor below the bedrooms, so I could relieve myself without worrying that someone would hear me or wonder why I was taking so long.

On the following day we traveled to our final destination, a campsite in the south of France. The bathroom situation at the campsite was pretty bad. We were in a small caravan with basically cardboard for walls, so you might as well have asked me to poop in the village square. I achieved my constipation record on this holiday: four and a half days without a bowel movement, which is probably not that long to a normal person, but for my sensitive guts it meant guaranteed pain.

Perhaps the worst moment of the trip took place on a boat. We had booked a short trip to explore the coast on the sort of small speedboat that you find in tourist destinations. Once we were out of the harbor, the sea became quite rough and at one point we all got soaked. There was no danger though. Everyone was laughing and it was all very exciting, and without the IBS it would have been great. With the IBS it was just depressing, thinking about how much fun I would have been having if my stomach hadn't felt like lead.

I am sure that my friend ended up thinking that she had badly misjudged me. I was a good friend at school and the greatest grump imaginable when on holiday. But it was almost impossible to act normally when my stomach was killing me, let alone act like I was having the time of my life. In fact, the acting can be one of the most demoralizing things about this condition. If there's anything more tiring, more soul-destroying, than pretending to be happy, I don't know what it might be.

Another memory involves a camping trip to Wales where I became predictably constipated and then had a wonderfully entertaining bathroom session. I have few memories of the fun parts of the trip, but extremely detailed memories of sitting in a tent playing cards and desperately trying to act like I was having fun while my guts tried to eat me from the inside.

And it wasn't just constipation and pain. I also suffered from a bloated feeling, like my stomach was being inflated with a bicycle pump. Plus, my intestines were so sensitive I could almost *feel* food moving through my gut. On the days when I was "just" constipated, it would feel like someone was stretching my stomach continuously, as if a gripping, grinning gremlin was constantly prodding me in the side.

I began to develop the ability to interpret my stomach like a pro. Is it a minor, five-second pain caused by gas? That'll normally be a kind of stretching, sharpish pain that will diminish pretty quickly. Is it an unremitting, right-hand side pain that feels like someone is squeezing my duodenum? That'll last for the whole day but may be relieved tomorrow morning. Is it an explosion of pain that makes me sweat and grit my teeth? That'll need a bathroom for an hour and then things will get back to normal.

On top of all this was the physical aspect of dealing with diarrhea. I would sometimes have to strip, wash myself and get dressed again. Like a teenage version of a two-year-old, except that two-year-olds get to grow out of it.

CHAPTER 2

Surviving School and University

A PREDICTABLE PATTERN OF SYMPTOMS HAD BEEN SET, which continued throughout my school years from ages 12 to 18. I would often be constipated and when I was constipated I was usually in pain. From time to time, an attack of diarrhea would relieve the pain, but the constipation would soon return.

When I was about 15, I began to think that I might have IBS. I hadn't seen a doctor yet, and I wouldn't receive a proper diagnosis from a doctor until many years later. In the meantime, I decided I needed to do my own research.

I can't remember where I heard the name IBS. This was before the invention of the Internet, so I couldn't diagnose myself with a quick Google. So I bought a book about IBS and turned straight to the section that listed the symptoms of an irritable bowel. And there I was in black and white: diarrhea, constipation, stomach pain and bloating. The authors even said that many sufferers dated their symptoms back to an attack of food poisoning.

The book also described the Manning Criteria, a complete list of symptoms that you could expect to find in an IBS patient. These criteria have been replaced in recent years by the Rome Criteria, but the symptom list remains roughly the same. If I had three or more of the following symptoms, plus abdominal pain, then I was a candidate for IBS:

- pain relieved by defecation
- more frequent stools with pain onset
- looser stools with pain onset
- abdominal distension
- mucus in the stool
- a feeling of incomplete evacuation after defecation

I definitely had abdominal pain, and it usually went away when I was able to have a bowel movement or five. The most intense pain was always linked to frequent stools. I felt bloated and, although I hadn't gone so far as to measure my waistline, I thought that "abdominal distension" was probably in the bag too. So that was three symptoms plus abdominal pain. It sounded like I might have IBS.

But self-diagnosing by using the above list is not a wise thing to do. The Manning Criteria had the significant caveat that IBS could only be diagnosed if your symptoms matched the list and there was *an absence of other bowel diseases,* which meant that the symptoms I was experiencing could have indicated anything from colitis to bowel cancer.

It probably goes without saying that I wasn't particularly thrilled about the possibility of having IBS. I would have thought that one of the most important rules for choosing a new illness is not to pick one with the word *bowel* in the title. In many ways, though, the name didn't matter. It was already apparent that I didn't have a nice, polite, genteel condition where I could look a bit pale and cough quietly into my handkerchief. I had a bowel problem and you can't make that sound pretty, whatever its name.

The rest of my new book was not very reassuring. It said no one knew what caused IBS, there was no cure, and many doctors did not take it seriously, despite the fact that it could ruin patients' lives. Many of the chapters described treatments for IBS, but there seemed to be little consensus as to which treatments actually worked. There were so many different pills and potions and therapies and theories that I didn't know where to start. I wanted a little flowchart that read, "Get IBS—get drugs—get cured," but that was a long way from the reality. I would later realize that it's a bad idea to suffer from any medical condition that has 200 treatments; the best diseases have a solution that works for everyone.

The book also included quotes from other IBS sufferers, which were half comforting (I was clearly not alone) and half horrifying (other people's symptoms were much worse than mine). One sufferer said, "I cope very badly. I'm in tears most days as it's so bad when I get up and continues through the day and night." Another said, "I feel that four years out of the five I've had IBS have been ruined, wasted." Still another: "I get so depressed and fed up with myself because it's not fair to my son to find me in bed all the time when he gets home from school."

This was not good news.

In the face of all this new information, I decided it was time to seek medical help, so I summoned up the courage to go to the doctor for the first time. The doctor listened to me describe my symptoms for a few minutes, prescribed some senna laxative pills, and sent me home. He didn't mention IBS or any other possible diagnosis, and I think he assumed that I had a boring old case of constipation.

This was the first time I had ever discussed my symptoms out loud, and it was mortifying. I remember saying that I had difficulty going to the toilet and then having to clarify that I meant bowel movements rather than peeing. The doctor said something like, "And what would you like me to do about that?" I think he must have been asking whether I had a specific treatment in mind, rather than saying, "Leave my office at once you lying malingerer." Nevertheless, it wasn't very comforting at the time.

He gave me the laxatives without further advice, and I felt that he hadn't been overly supportive or interested in my case. Plus, the embarrassment of picking up the laxatives from the chemist had almost killed me. I had sat in the chemist waiting for the assistant to call my name, silently urging her not to read out any labels in my general direction. Of course, chemists give out all kinds of embarrassing things, and I doubt they call out, "Penis pump for Mr. Stanford," but that didn't stop me worrying.

So my first foray into the medical world was really rather useless, and I was still struggling with all the same symptoms. The most miserable times were when the IBS would spoil a special day or event that I knew would otherwise have been fantastic. Day-to-day school wasn't that much of a problem, because if one day was spoilt then there was always another one just like it. But when it's a day that you'll never get back, it's depressing.

On the day of a school trip to a theme park I woke up, had my breakfast and couldn't go to the bathroom for the life of me. If I can't go in the morning, it's a guarantee that I won't be able to go for the rest of the day. I had to face hours and hours of watching my friends having fun while pretending that my stomach wasn't killing me.

It seemed like such a stupid reason to be miserable. I wasn't dying, my limbs weren't broken. Even when I was constipated, I often felt okay: not great, but not terrible, either. But there was always that tightness to my stomach and that uncomfortable, stretched, bloated feeling to remind me that my body wasn't working properly. These feelings made it impossible to relax.

Despite all of this, my IBS was pretty manageable during my school days, for which I am grateful. For example, I often managed 100 percent attendance for the school year, not taking a single day off sick. I was in the orchestra and choir and took flute and piano lessons. I was a prefect and got good grades and passed my exams and had fun with my friends. I had some very bad times, but I also had plenty of days when I felt fine. The worst times were yet to come.

University

As I reached the age of 18, my friends started to plan their futures. Most were going on to university and I had decided to do the same, with some trepidation at the thought of being in a strange place with strange people and a bowel that didn't work. I had applied to study English and American Literature because I was a bit of a book nerd and English had always been my best subject.

Of all the students in the country, worrying about their social lives and academic lives and debt, I imagined that I was the only one worrying about her bowels.

Even applying to university was stressful, and the interview process for one university was utterly terrifying. I had to go and stay in a residence hall for two whole nights. During the time I was there, I had to sit for an exam and then have two interviews with professors who had intelligence pouring out of them and smoked and stared at the ceiling, bored out of their minds, while I blathered on about poetry. Thankfully, my bowel decided to co-operate, and I was not required to ask the scariest people I had ever seen in my life if they would mind waiting while I practiced my pooping skills.

I was finally accepted at Warwick University—a school that didn't interview prospective students. The city of Coventry, where Warwick University is based, was about two and a half hours away by car, so that meant moving away from home completely and living with a hundred or so students I had never met.

This was daunting enough by itself, but people kept saying to me, "Oh well, everyone will be in the same situation, won't they? They'll be just as nervous as you."

They might be just as nervous, I thought, *but at least they had mastered the art of digestion.*

In my first year at university I had a room in one of the residence halls on campus. There were a few rooms on campus that had en suite bathrooms, but they were much more expensive than a standard room and very difficult to get. I hadn't really tried to get one either, although I'm not sure why. I suppose I thought that the communal bathrooms were going to come with a little more privacy than they actually did.

All of the halls of residence had different versions of a shared bathroom setup. Some bathrooms were completely separate toilets in their own room, like you would find in many homes, shared between four or five students. Other bathrooms were the kind of open-plan, three toilets strung together arrangements that you might find in a shopping center, the ones that let everyone know exactly what you are doing and why.

There were three toilets on my floor, for about twelve people, which is an okay ratio, but it wasn't an okay situation. The problem was that the toilets were anything but private. There were gaps underneath the doors the size of wildebeest and gaps at the tops of the doors as well. There were showers in the same room as the toilets so there was no privacy to speak of. You even had to worry about the cleaners, who came around every morning as regular as clockwork to polish things and tidy up.

This was all pretty alarming. I had to stay in the halls until the end of my first year, when students moved off campus into rented houses. How was I going to cope without becoming a laughing stock, "that girl who lives in the loos"?

This might all sound like ridiculous paranoia. But IBS had made me very self-conscious about my bodily functions, and no wonder. I quickly learned that these subjects don't seem to generate a lot of sympathy, and sufferers are much more likely to be greeted with laughter than with empathy. By this time, I had been suffering from IBS for six years. I don't think it's unreasonable for me to have developed a bit of a bathroom phobia during that time, or at least a phobia about other people's reactions to my bathroom habits. My bathroom habits were many and varied and often deeply, deeply strange.

In the end, my first year at university was not that bad. I still struggled with constipation and its fellow symptoms, but for the most part I was able to carry on as normal and keep up with my work and even manage a semblance of a social life.

Within my hall of residence, though, I had managed to keep my secret rather too well. No one in my hall knew that I had IBS, but no one really knew *me* either. If I met someone in the corridors I would often try to avoid speaking to them. Under no circumstances did I want to be having a friendly chat with someone right before we both went into the bathroom and I had to demonstrate my IBS bowel.

In my second year, I arranged to move into a student house with a group of friends. We had visited our prospective house while I was still living on campus, just to check that it wasn't the black hole of Calcutta. It was quite nice, as student houses go. It had five bedrooms, two toilets and a garden, and although it was quite small, it seemed to be decent enough.

The main bathroom was particularly interesting, because it had a sliding wooden door. The reason for the sliding door was, I think, that the bathroom was right at the top of the stairs, so any door that stuck out onto the landing would have been a safety hazard. Oddly enough, I didn't take much notice of the sliding door when I first saw the house. My main thought was that it was great to have an extra loo downstairs, so if someone was in the main bathroom when I had an IBS attack I was not going to have to wait in pain.

When we moved in, however, I began to spot the problem with the door. Your average hinge-reliant door tends to make a fairly good seal with the door frame, and therefore acts as a decent sound barrier. Your sliding door does not.

Another problem was that it didn't really lock properly. We agreed that whenever the door was pulled across it was not to be opened from the outside, but it still meant that any half-asleep housemate could walk in on you if they'd forgotten that the lock didn't work.

In addition, the walls of the bathroom were paper-thin, which meant that anyone within ten feet of the room gained a really clear idea of my efforts inside.

Toilet break

You may be wondering at this point why on earth I was so obsessed with toilets. Well, because that's what IBS did to me, I'm afraid. Imagine something worse than messing your pants in public. What did you pick? Being flayed and burnt alive? Having an aardvark forever up your nose?

There really can't be anything more embarrassing than the prospect of fecal incontinence; even the name is disgusting. And at other times I found that if I did not heed my body's warning to go to the toilet *right this minute,* my intestines would go on strike for the rest of the day.

My guts, if they are working at all, are programmed to go to the loo about half an hour to an hour after breakfast. If I miss that perfect time slot, I'll be in for some pretty serious discomfort. If someone's in the bathroom when I'm dying to go, or I just can't get to a loo, then I've just volunteered for some guaranteed pain.

At university I quickly scoped out the best and worst toilets on campus. There were various qualities that I looked for in a toilet, with privacy being the most important. My dream toilet would be soundproof, hidden away in a quiet corner, and unavailable to anyone but me.

If you happen to find yourself on campus at Warwick University then here are my toilet recommendations.

Main library toilets (English literature section)—very useful and private, often empty, especially on weekends. Runner-up position in the toilet competition.

Computer room toilets—situated just around the corner from one of the student computer rooms, these were some of my favorite loos on the whole of the campus. There were only two cubicles so I would often have the entire bathroom to myself, or if I didn't, I could wait for the other cubicle to empty before doing my thing, as long as my bowel would cooperate.

Not many people even seemed to know that this bathroom existed, as it was nicely tucked away and not well sign-posted. It was also very conveniently placed, halfway between my hall of residence and the English literature classrooms. Very highly recommended.

Westwood music room toilets—Westwood was a mini campus mainly for postgraduates, and it happened to be where my hall of residence was located. There was a music department building there with practice rooms and piano rooms, and most of the time, especially in the evenings, it was deserted. More importantly, its loos were deserted too. I spent some very happy times in this toilet.

So as you can see, toilets are very important to me. The first time I got my own flat the thing that I was most pleased about was the fact that I had a toilet to call my own. It's true.

* * *

In the end, things weren't as bad as I had expected with that sliding door in my shared student house. My big advantage was that I was an English literature student while the rest of my housemates were doing proper courses where you actually had to go to lectures rather than read books all the time, so I often had the house to myself.

It wasn't an ideal situation, but in some ways it was better than my first year in the hall of residence. At least now there were times when I had a bathroom all to myself, and my housemates were the nicest people in the whole world so I thought that if I ever did have a massively loud and epic IBS attack they probably wouldn't fall about laughing.

However, I was still suffering on a regular basis. I spent an awful lot of lectures and seminars nursing a painful stomach and a blocked bowel. I'd tried a couple of different laxatives by then, bought furtively from the local chemist, and they usually cleared me out. But they often caused extra pain as well and they only ever worked for one day. By the next morning I would be constipated again.

I could have tried taking a laxative every night, but I could slip over into diarrhea so easily that this didn't seem like a good idea, and I was also worried about making my bowel even more dysfunctional through over-medication.

At one point, I decided to take a slightly different approach. One of the key problems was that if I was unable to have a bowel movement in the morning then I was usually blocked up for the whole day and relief would only come the next morning, either naturally or via a laxative.

I needed something that would work immediately or within a few minutes. There seemed to be two basic options for this: suppositories or enemas. I suppose that colon hydrotherapy or colonics would have qualified as options as well, but I didn't really fancy lying on a table half naked while some stranger rammed a tube up my bottom and gave it a good spring clean.

Enemas seemed to be almost as off-putting as hydrotherapy, just being a smaller, home-based version of the tube-up-the-bottom routine, so that left suppositories. I plucked up my courage and went suppository shopping.

The tried-and-tested way to buy these things is to fill your basket with a plethora of non-embarrassing stuff and hope that no one notices the enemas and hemorrhoid cream, so that's what I did. I just about survived it. (Of course the miracle of the Internet now allows people to buy everything from suppositories to mini condoms in blissful anonymity.)

So I was now in proud possession of some glycerin suppositories, which looked rather like little torpedoes made out of firm gel. The idea was to simply insert the suppository into my backside, wait ten or fifteen minutes for the gel stuff to stimulate the muscles of the colon, and then have an easy bowel movement.

Or that's what was supposed to happen. What actually happened was that I inserted the suppository, waited five minutes, felt like I really, really had to go to the loo right away, went to the loo, and pooped out a remarkably well-formed suppository. The suppository had successfully induced an urge to poop, therefore, but only to poop itself. It was a self-referential, post-modern suppository, and I was as blocked up as ever.

CHAPTER 3

My Diary

IN MY THIRD YEAR AT UNIVERSITY I STARTED TO KEEP A DIARY. It was not meant to be a bowel diary specifically, but inevitably a lot of the entries mentioned my intestinal struggles.

I have included some excerpts from my diary in this chapter to show my day-to-day battle with my digestion. I used the word "bobbed" to stand for constipated/in pain/general IBS problems. It stood for "Blocked of Bowel," which I think was my attempt to make something disgusting and painful sound cute and fluffy.

Bear in mind that at this stage in my life the IBS was still a closely guarded secret. I hadn't yet told anyone that I was a sufferer, not even my parents, and I really didn't plan to talk about it at all if I didn't have to.

24 August 1998

Went to Matt's for his 21st birthday party. Went to music store and got some new stuff, including Tom Lehrer book. Favorite line: "Soon we'll be sliding down the razor blade of life."

Went back to Matt's house and did present-giving and slept on lounge floor. Saw a movie on Sunday, when bobbed as expected. Depressing week of bobbing subsequently, in no mood to record my profundities for posterity.

1 September 1998

Having a difficult time bowel-wise. Wonder what I'll think looking back on this in 10 years' time. Hope bowel has got its bloody act together by then.

16 September 1998

Went to the Last Night of the Proms concert, or rather Proms in the Park. Felt good.

Sunday was less good for usual away-from-home reason (bobbed). Then yesterday evening Matt calls me to say he was dismayed that we don't seem to be picking our friendship up from where we left off in term time.

Really had no idea what he meant, Saturday was great, I thought everything was fine apart from my rather abrupt departure on Sunday, but then I had a good reason for that.

After visiting my friend for a few days, I had left his house on a Sunday afternoon, announcing pretty much out of nowhere that I wanted to go home. My friend had been understandably baffled by my behavior, being as I was all smiley and happy on Saturday and then sullen and withdrawn just one day later.

I say in the diary that I had a good reason for my "abrupt departure," but had I told my friend what it was? Nope. All I had wanted to do was go home and try to sort out my beleaguered bowel, to be somewhere where I didn't have to pretend to be sociable and healthy. But the trouble was that if I didn't actually tell people what was wrong—and I didn't because of the very nature of IBS—they started thinking that I was bored with them or disliked them because I was so often running away.

19 September 1998

Declaring war on bowel with help of Good Health magazine. Sick to death of the whole bloody business.

24 September 1998

Am happy and bowel is functioning. Little things for little minds. Wonder if anyone else records the habits of their colon in diary form. Suspect not.

29 October 1998

Went to concert last night which was great, but spoiled by bowel. Basically life is great if only my bowel would comply. Hoping for doctor's miracle tomorrow.

2 November 1998

Doctor has given me some Fybogel stuff to try. Is orange and doesn't taste too bad. Have three months' supply, so here's hoping. Doctor was quite nice, but at one point said re: bowel problems: "And how does that bother you?" You try it, mate. Didn't say that of course.

The doctor had also prescribed Lactulose, which is an osmotic laxative: that is, it draws water into the bowel to make the stool softer and looser. It comes in the form of a very sweet syrup that is tasty and nauseating at the same time. It seemed to help a little, but as usual it was not the whole answer. The Fybogel was a similar story, perhaps taking the edge off my symptoms but offering no real improvement beyond that.

I was also experimenting with a couple of other remedies. Linusit Gold linseed, known as flaxseed in some countries, is recommended in several IBS books as a way to increase fiber intake, and comes in the form of little seeds that are sprinkled on cereal or swallowed with water. It's very easy to take, tastes quite nice, and I got the pleasure of seeing some of the undigested seeds get passed several days later. But it didn't do much for my symptoms.

Then there was aloe vera, which in some forms can be a very potent laxative and in others is supposed to help calm the bowel. It seemed to help at first, despite its completely vile taste, but then it started giving me some fierce intestinal spasms. That was the end of that.

26 November 1998

Bloody awful day yesterday. Got up with pain in behind and feeling crappy (first day of period) and things just got worse from there, stomach-wise. Seems to be recurring thing on period now, oh joy.

Even healthy women can suffer from diarrhea or constipation as a normal part of their menstrual cycle, and these symptoms are usually blamed on hormonal fluctuations. IBS sufferers are even more susceptible to these variations.

I was used to fairly painful period cramps on their own, but combined with the pain of an IBS attack and the joys of diarrhea, my monthly cycle became something to dread. Some of my worst IBS attacks of all time have coincided with the first day of my period. These attacks would start off with intense pain, the worst I had ever felt in my life, combined with gut-wrenching intestinal spasms. I would get perhaps ten minutes' warning from my stomach and then I would have to use the toilet three or four times with breaks of between a few minutes and half an hour between each trip. During these breaks I would be literally writhing around in pain.

Sometimes I wouldn't even bother leaving the bathroom because the diarrhea was so severe. When these attacks happened all I could do was sit on the toilet sweating and shaking and waiting it out.

Immediately after an attack was over I would feel almost euphoric. I had survived another one! I wasn't going to be in agony for the rest of my life! I could leave the bathroom! But this euphoria would quickly fade as I realized that I had had yet another IBS attack, and they weren't going away any time soon.

12 December 1998

Bewitched, bobbed and bewildered. Always happens at the end of term–bowel gives up the ghost for the holidays and (break for sitting in car for hours).

3 January 1999

Am so sick of it. Knowing it will spoil every holiday, every weekend, every other bloody day. Damn it all to hell. Have just looked back through diary and there are so many bad days due to bowel, it's frightening. I must do something about it, there must be a solution somewhere. Probably not in melodrama. I'll keep going for want of a better plan.

7 January 1999

I AM SO STRESSED!! Really bloody stressed I am. Am trying to unbugger bowel via Internet. Am so sick of it, so sick of the pain and the struggling and the search for a cure.

Went to Matt's on Tuesday. Then Wednesday had normal blocked bowel and just wanted to get home. Have to be cheerful and normal though, that's the worst part. If I had "proper" illness or no right arm or something I'd get sympathy. As it is, I have to act perfectly bloody chirpy while feeling, literally, like crap.

Feel like a constipated hero, silent in her suffering. Just want it to stop so I can stress over something else for a change.

27 March 1999

Had an interview for postgraduate course. Had to get up at 6 a.m., travel to London, take the tube and find the place.

Had bizarre intestine spasms, due to eating breakfast so early I guess. Had to do written tests, then interview in the afternoon after having spent quarter of an hour in the toilet for lunch. Interview was OK though.

3 April 1999

Worrying about InterRailing. Ed has asked me go round Europe with him and a group of friends. Think it's a bad idea because of bowel. Is bound to play up and ruin it. Have said yes to him now though and figure my only real option is to tell him the truth about intestines.

7 April 1999

Have sent Ed an honest letter. Bit tense about it.

8 April 1999

Ed called and was remarkably cheerful and unfazed, so that's all dealt with. Bowel is extremely well today. Surely some mistake.

This was the first time in my life that I had told anyone apart from a doctor about my symptoms, and in some ways it was rather an anti-climax. My friend just rang me and we talked about the IBS for a while and that was that. He didn't laugh at me or flee in horror. I don't know quite what I had been expecting him to do, but I certainly hadn't expected him to be so, well, grown-up about the thing.

I should have learned a lot from this first utterance of the illness that dare not speak its name. I should have learned that people were not going to shun me because of it, that anyone who was a genuine friend was going to be understanding and try to help. Instead I breathed a sigh of relief and went straight back to suffering in silence.

Monday the something of something (lost track of time a bit here)

Have been invited to Kim's belated 21st birthday party, and am trying to come up with legitimate reasons not to go–cat died, dog ate my bus pass, had a stroke, that kind of thing.

Have no real social life beyond housemates, but then when I am invited to something sociable, I'd rather eat a wardrobe.

20 July 1999

Have had a bloody awful week, constipated every damn day. Felt like giving up, just giving up. Completely wasted week, wasted bloody years of my life just waiting for the next day.

1 August 1999

Feel like I've done nothing for the last three months. Must try harder. Have lost all semblance of self-discipline.

Understand that some of this is bowel-related. Going well at the moment, but is always hanging over my head (not good image).

4 January 2000

New Year's resolution–to make it through a whole term with no bobbing. That'll be a miracle. Was fine until Millennium Eve then it went haywire again because I got up late the next day.

Bloody hell. Very pissed off. As last year really. Nothing much changes. Just find something new to pin my fragile hopes to until it fails. Isn't life fun? Thought aloe vera was working, but it doesn't seem to cope with me getting up a bit late, very feeble effort.

Suppose should record Millennium Eve events for posterity, although seems ages ago now in blessed functioning bowel times of yore. Went to Tasha's for street party, lit lots of candles in jam jars, sang carols in the street, got a bit wet, almost got a bit dead from stray firework.

Very good night generally, paying for it now in the pleasure/pain life balance. Must cling to resolution.

Reading these old diary entries makes me pretty depressed. What they show is that I had a good life: nice friends, nice university, a nice student house. And a terrible irritable bowel. If only I had been able to find something to calm it down I would have had a much better time at university, but it just seemed to keep flaring up with no warning.

The length of time that I had been suffering from IBS was also beginning to really weigh me down. If you had offered me the choice, I think there's a good possibility that I would have asked to be in terrible pain for a day rather than moderate pain off and on for the rest of my life. If I'd known that I just had to survive another few months, even another few years with the pain, it might have been easier to cope. But there seemed to be no end in sight.

The diary also shows that I was terrible at communicating with my friends when it came to IBS. I only told one friend about it the whole time I was at university and that was only because I was practically forced into it as he had invited me on holiday and there's no way that my bowel would have coped. I am sure that this secretive attitude hurt my friendships.

You end up making excuses for things and acting strangely because you are trying to live your life around the IBS, but if your friends don't know that the IBS is there then it must be like watching someone play chess with an invisible frog, just incomprehensibly odd.

And when the IBS was rampant, my behavior must have seemed even more bizarre. At one stage, an old school friend invited me to come and stay with her for the weekend. This would involve just one overnight stay, and therefore only one morning away from my home toilet, and so I went. And I just about managed it. Except for a tight-feeling stomach, it wasn't too bad.

Things got a lot worse when I returned the invitation and invited her to stay with me for the weekend. I woke up on the Saturday and found myself constipated, so I had to go to the train station to pick her up with my best acting face on and make sure she knew I was happy to see her. Once I had brought her back to my house, my bowel promptly woke up, so I had to leave her alone in my room while my intestines emptied themselves.

Then in the evening we went out for a pizza. My bowel decided that this would be another good time to expel its wares, so I had to leave her again while I went to the pizza place toilet and had another IBS session.

On Sunday, things were even more exciting. We went into town and did some window shopping. It was absolutely totally freezing cold and carrying on from the night before, my IBS was now in full-on diarrhea mode. As it was Sunday, there weren't many shops open, and nowhere with a bathroom. Even if a toilet had been available, my bowel felt so bad that I thought I might go into the bathroom and never be able to leave, abandoning my friend in an unfamiliar town on a freezing cold Sunday with no explanation whatsoever. In the end my rumbling guts calmed down enough for me to get home. Of course, by the time I got to a toilet I didn't need to go anymore.

The entire weekend was a veritable showcase for the wide range of intestinal delights that my body was able to produce, and I spent most of it either running to the bathroom or trying—and failing—to concentrate on something other than the state of my digestion.

CHAPTER 4

IBS Experiences Around the World

FOR A REASON THAT NOW ESCAPES ME I agreed, while still at university, to go on a choir trip. We would travel by coach to the Czech Republic and Hungary, singing at various cathedrals and venues along the way.

In practical terms, this meant that I would be sitting on a coach for around sixteen hours to get to our first destination and later for shorter periods of time as we traveled from place to place. It would also mean two-hour concerts, foreign and unusual food, and no time alone to sit and nurse my stomach.

God knows what I was thinking. I suppose it was something along the lines of *I would very much like to have fun with my friends and sing some songs, and I shall pretend that my bowel will let me.* So off I went.

The coach journey itself was fairly uneventful. One "advantage" of having IBS with more constipation than diarrhea was that I could sit on a coach for sixteen hours and not be ridiculously worried about the toilet situation.

Once we got to the hotel I was definitely worried about the toilet situation. There was one large bathroom for each floor of the hotel, and our bathroom contained three showers and three toilet cubicles. One of the toilets had no door, one had no lock, and one had no toilet.

Just as an extra bonus, the showers were completely open-plan, and I mean *completely* open-plan. You could walk into the bathroom and get a very good view of whoever happened to be showering at the time, as well as anyone who had chosen the toilet with no front door. I didn't have a body phobia as much as a bowel phobia, but I wasn't that thrilled about flashing my bits to all and sundry. The whole setup was far from ideal.

Of course, we didn't stay in the hotel all the time. The whole point of the trip was to sing in front of European audiences, and we also had various excursions arranged so that we could see different places of interest and do some touristy things.

On one of these excursions, a trip to a Hungarian city, my friend and I were walking along a backstreet when I felt the need for a loo. And the need for a loo became a pressing need for a loo, and a pressing need for a loo became a find-me-a-toilet-right-now-or-we're-all-going-to-be-very-very-sorry situation. I had no idea whether Hungary had public toilets, and if it did whether you had to pay for them or if they were a hole in the ground or a bucket in a hut or who knows what. I had no idea what to do.

So I waited, clenching my buttocks carefully, and hoped the urge would go away. And it did! Thank the good gut Lord for that. At least until we were at the concert venue and getting changed into our choir clothes backstage, when the urge decided to come back, bless its heart. I was now in a slightly better situation than before, but not by much. There were about twelve of us getting changed in the same room, and the toilet was sort of en suite. It was practically *in* the room, shoved up in one corner as if it had been a cupboard in a previous life. Now, granted, there was a door and even a lock on this one, but it was still a bit intimidating.

Not only that, but because we were going to be singing for the next couple of hours everyone wanted to go to the loo beforehand. So there was a nice long polite British queue, and a guarantee that someone would use the loo directly after me, just after I had released the torrent of whatever nasty old thing inside me had been trying to escape all day.

But what can you do? I went to the bathroom, my intestines exploded (luckily quite quietly and neatly), I flushed the toilet and hoped for the best in regards to smells and mess.

There is one other memory of this trip that is very firmly lodged in my mind. We were on the underground train somewhere in the Czech Republic. It was quite crowded and I was standing next to a man and a woman who had their arms around each other. They were just about the most glamorous pair of people I have ever seen in my life. The man was dark and handsome, and very well dressed, and the woman was beautiful. They looked like they'd stepped out of a perfume commercial.

I, on the other hand, hadn't been to the bathroom for several days, and my protesting intestines chose to register their disapproval by releasing a smell that could have felled a full-grown yak. I will always remember the sight of that beautiful girl looking at me from her boyfriend's arms and wrinkling her nose in disgust.

This was how it would be. Other people would be beautiful, loved and healthy, and I would fart on trains.

Graduation

I got myself through the rest of my time at university, avoiding any more foreign exploits. My symptoms remained much the same, and they were always manageable but draining. I didn't have any horrific IBS accidents in the middle of the students' union, and I didn't have symptoms that were so bad they stopped me from studying or having fun, but they were enough to put a big black cloud over my life and to always remind me that I was an IBS sufferer.

I also had ongoing problems staying away from home, as any kind of trip or even the shortest overnight stay seemed to throw my bowels into chaos. By this time I had accumulated a long list of holidays and trips that my bowel had decided to spoil.

Just to add to the fun, the human mind is programmed to clearly remember anything that is particularly emotional or intense, and so I found that I was often left with a wonderfully vivid memory of some of the most difficult days of my life. I have a very special file in my brain marked *IBS Experiences to Treasure.* Here are some of my favorite examples:

Four Weddings and a Funeral—I saw this film at a small cinema in Wales when I was on a camping holiday with two of my friends. I was very constipated and my stomach was bloated and painful. I didn't think the film was as good as people had been saying, although I do now, having seen it without the pain filter.

New Year's Eve—I'm in London, standing beneath Big Ben. There is a crowd of people, laughing and singing, surrounding me. I am there with my friend, and we have been in several pubs and had several drinks. My intestines are not enjoying themselves.

The Reduced Shakespeare Company Short History of America—you may have heard of the Reduced Shakespeare Company theater group. They basically take something huge like the complete works of Shakespeare (hence the name) or the entire history of America and condense it into a two-hour comedy show.

I had gone to stay with my friend in London, and by the time I saw this show I had already been there for two nights. My bowels had entirely shut up shop and would remain completely blocked for the duration of my four-day stay. I couldn't take a laxative because we were sightseeing and getting out and about and enjoying ourselves. Plus, I didn't want to poop in St. Paul's Cathedral.

The previous night, by which time I was already in pain, we had seen the musical *Fame*. I don't remember much about the show except wishing I was someone else in the audience because they all seemed to be having so much fun. By the time I got to see the Reduced Shakespeare Company I just wanted to go home and go to bed.

While most of my symptoms were very much part of the established pattern of pain, constipation and diarrhea, there was one incident that had been really unusual. During one toilet visit, part of a constipation cycle where I had been straining away to try to gain victory over a particularly intransigent bowel movement, I had noticed some bright red blood on the toilet paper. It seemed obvious to me at the time that this was caused by breaking a few blood vessels due to all of the straining. In other words, I had hemorrhoids.

There wasn't a huge amount of blood, and it only appeared for that one toilet visit, so I wasn't particularly concerned about it. It didn't seem like much to worry about in comparison with the rest of the symptoms I was experiencing.

This is yet another little incident under the *Do as I say and not as I do* heading, because bleeding is a so-called "red flag" symptom when it comes to irritable bowel syndrome, a symptom that should be investigated by a doctor since it is not characteristic of IBS. I should have gone to the doctor's office, but I didn't. Luckily it turned out to be just a hemorrhoid, but it still wasn't the brightest decision I ever made.

My little hemorrhoid proved to be a minor distraction from my usual IBS-soaked life, which was now moving on. After graduation I went on to do a postgraduate journalism course at Cardiff University in Wales. I'd decided to do journalism as I enjoyed writing and it seemed like a natural progression from the English degree.

I rented a little bedsit in a tree-lined street in Cardiff, and luckily my living arrangements came with a bit more privacy this time. Although the bathrooms were still shared, there were two toilets for six people, and neither toilet was right next to anyone's bedroom or behind a sliding door.

I was even less inclined to tell my fellow students about the IBS though, as they were all very confident, competent people. I couldn't imagine any of them with diarrhea problems and bloated colons. In reality, by the law of averages I expect at least a few of them sometimes had colon problems, but I would never have found out because it's not polite to talk about intestines.

So once again, I mostly kept myself to myself, did my work, went to as few pub outings as possible and just got on with the basic stuff of living, going to school and graduating. I could have been having a much better time.

My symptoms remained boringly predictable. My bowel would shut down at the drop of a hat and would occasionally have a major clean-out just for fun. Any unusual event such as getting up at 5:30 a.m. for one London journalism conference would put my bowel into such a huff that it would keep me in pain throughout the day.

I would be happily enjoying my life, doing my work and getting on with everything, when the IBS would completely take over. It was rather like my daily cycle into university, a lovely route across a park. The entrance to the park was right next to a busy road and every morning I'd be cycling along thinking what a lovely morning it was when I'd spot two or three dead hedgehogs in the gutter. That was my life: good things and happiness and friendship and fun and dead hedgehog dead hedgehog dead hedgehog.

The journalism course only lasted for one academic year, so before I knew it I was out in the real world looking for a job. This worried me. Doing a student course was one thing, but a nine-to-five job was something different altogether. The postgraduate course had been hard work, but I often took time off to study, plus weekends and long holidays.

The only time I had worked consistently in a full-time job was one summer break when I worked for about ten weeks as an admin assistant in my dad's office. I'd had to go into work a couple of times feeling rough. There had been one day when I'd spent the whole lunch hour in the loo to ease my terrible stomach cramps, but I had managed it.

But that had been a ten-week thing. If I got a full-time job I was going to have to work nine-to-five, five days a week, forever and ever. And I had no idea whether I could cope.

There was nothing else for it though. I had no trust fund to live off, and the days when I could just marry a passing rich man and live in his castle were long gone. Besides, castle bathrooms are notoriously chilly.

So I started applying for jobs. I had a couple of interviews and got nowhere, but then I was interviewed for a job with a sweet little publishing company that had an office very close to my undergraduate university. The job involved writing articles, proofreading books and generally helping out with the editorial side of things. On the day of the interview I had quite bad IBS symptoms and felt rather grim, but I pretended to be fine, and I was offered the job.

I would work fifty-two weeks a year with twenty days' holiday, seven hours a day in set hours. Just the standard stuff, and in our workaholic culture, this was really the minimum that anyone could get away with, but it was still a daunting prospect.

I knew that if I was ill one day I would just have to get on with it, even if I was still ill the next day and the next. I also knew that if I started taking time off from work then I was not going to be popular.

I suppose I could have been honest with my boss right from the start, but because that would probably have involved a teeth-grindingly embarrassing conversation about my symptoms, I kept quiet.

I also kept quiet because at this point I didn't really believe that I deserved special treatment for an irritable bowel. I didn't give myself enough credit as someone who was genuinely ill, as I just didn't see myself as someone with a long-term, chronic medical condition.

IBS comes and goes, waxes and wanes. Sometimes I felt really ill and sometimes I felt completely, totally healthy. It felt strange to think of myself as an ill person when some of the time, maybe as much as half of the time, I felt entirely well. But that means I felt ill for half the time that I was awake, and that's not normal, is it?

I suppose I hadn't come to terms with the fact that I was someone with quite a significant medical problem. It would be a while before I would accept this fact.

In the meantime, though, I had to face the first full-time job of my life, and I was scared. But I did draw some strength from the fact that I had always survived in the past. If I could get through a degree and a postgraduate course, surely I could cope with a job. Right?

CHAPTER 5

Finally Seeing a Gastroenterologist

I STARTED WORK AT THE SWEET LITTLE PUBLISHING COMPANY and almost immediately ran into trouble. The work was good and the people were lovely, but my IBS was getting worse and worse. In the past, I had always had time off from my IBS, periods of time when I felt normal and could forget about my problems for a while. This holiday time disappeared when I started my new job, and I began to feel pain every day, all day.

I'd rented a two-bedroom flat from one of my new colleagues, and he had been kind enough to let me have it for a very modest rate. So I was living in a large flat in the nicest block I'd ever lived in, with a brand-new job, and money in the bank, and my very own toilet. I was 22, with my whole life ahead of me, and I was drowning.

Sometimes I would sit at my desk and feel huge, horrible spasms run through my gut. It would be all I could do to keep sitting there. I would get myself through the day and then go home and collapse with a heating pad, hoping I would be better in the morning. I often wasn't.

It was so exhausting to be in pain all the time. Perhaps even more tiring was the fact that I had to pretend to be okay for work, struggling in every day without ever calling in sick. This may sound ridiculous to some people, especially those who don't have IBS. After all, if I was feeling ill then why didn't I take some time off?

Well, because that approach only works for normal illnesses. Your average person gets ill, gets better, and gets back to work. I get ill, stay ill, get a bit better, get ill again, stay ill, cry, maybe get a bit better if I'm lucky, and that's it. If I'd taken time off every time I felt bad, I would hardly ever have gone to work. And so my only options were to go to work and pretend to be okay, or to stay at home for literally months at a time.

On probably my worst day ever it actually felt like someone was stabbing me in the side every two minutes, over and over and over again, from eleven in the morning until nine at night. I sat at my desk clenching my fist and gritting my teeth to get through it.

Looking back, I probably should at least have taken *that* day off, but I told myself that I was saving my sick days up for when I felt really bad. I'm not quite sure how sick I thought I had to get before I deserved a sick day. Perhaps if my head had fallen off I would have taken an afternoon. It seems like crazy, self-destructive martyrdom now, but I guess I thought that if I started taking time off then I would never be able to stop.

There was another memorable day when I got up, pooped my pants in the living room, cleaned myself up, got dressed and went to work. How was I expected to live like this? I felt so far from normal I didn't know if I could ever make it back.

I had been in my job for four months when I was finally able to take a break and go home to my parents' house for the Christmas holidays. But I took the IBS home with me, so the break didn't do me much good. When I returned to my flat in the New Year, I found that the boiler had broken down and there was no central heating or hot water.

My wonderful parents went to the shops to buy me a couple of portable heaters, but to be honest I didn't really care about the cold. When my mum and dad left I sat on the floor, cross-legged, right in front of the TV, put my coat on and turned off all the heaters.

God knows why. I wasn't trying to get pneumonia, but it seemed like everything in my life was such an effort, even just keeping warm. If I could stop trying so hard, just sit on the floor and watch telly with my coat on forever and ever, then maybe I would be able to survive. But I couldn't, of course, and didn't. The next day I went back to work and arranged to get the boiler fixed and carried on carrying on.

The constant fight against this new severe version of IBS began to make me resentful and bitter. I spent one morning sitting and writing out a long list of my complaints against the world and my bowel, venting out all my anger against the constant discomfort that I was expected to simply live with.

On top of all this, I soon developed a brand spanking new health problem—back pain. For the last four months at work I had unwittingly been sitting on a chair that was very bad for my back. When I looked at it properly, I realized that it had basically no support for my lower back at all, and I had been stuck in it for at least seven hours each day.

And so my back had started to ache. Badly. This was all I needed. I came home after the first day of backache and burst into tears. I couldn't deal with a broken gut and now I had a broken back as well. How was I going to cope?

I decided to see a doctor about my backache, although I didn't hold out much hope. Doctors had always been civil to me, but not once had they really helped.

When I told the doctor about my back problem he asked me to bend over and touch my toes. He then said that I had a curved spine, that it was called kyphoscoliosis, and that swimming might help, but I shouldn't be too concerned about it, it wasn't as if my spine was crumbling away.

And that was that. It was rather like going to the doctor for bowel problems. You get prodded, patronized and sent home with no help. Do people go to the doctor and actually get their problems treated? Surely not. (I actually went to this doctor just once to talk about my bowel problems, and he asked me whether there had ever been problems with my toilet training; the implication being, of course, that overzealous or inadequate toilet training had caused years of irritable bowels. I sat there and gaped at him, which I'm sure was the appropriate response.)

Back at home, I tried to work out how crooked my back really was. Looking at my posture in the mirror I realized that not only was I slightly lopsided in my hips, I also had a fairly pronounced curve at the top of my spine that made me look a little slumped over, even when I was standing up straight.

Fantastic, I thought. I was a constipated, bloated, intestinally demented young hunchback. I prepared for the influx of suitors.

Lonely Hearts Advert

Young professional female, brown hair, blue eyes, often constipated, seeks deformed man who likes staying in and listening to people moan about their bowels. Must have own bathroom.

Giving in

I couldn't cope anymore. I was exhausted, in pain, and the only people I could confide in were my parents. I had finally owned up to them about the IBS in an e-mail, and they had been amazed that I had suffered for so long without telling them.

I was crying every single day, and it felt like an enormous effort just to get up in the morning and breathe. So, feeling very pathetic and weak, after only four months in my job, I collapsed in a little sobbing heap in the corner of my flat. It was a Sunday evening, and the thought of getting through another week at work was completely impossible. I was still in my pajamas and dressing gown because even getting dressed was too much for me.

I called my dad, broke down in tears and asked him to come and rescue me. I am very lucky to have a terrific family, and my dad drove for two and a half hours to pick me up the next day and take me home with him. I remember sitting in the car crying on the way home, feeling like a total failure. What kind of person couldn't even survive a few months of full-time work? Well, I try to be less hard on myself now—an IBS person, that's who! No one should be expected to work full-time when they are feeling so ill so often, but at the time it just felt like defeat.

Back at home with my parents, I was miserable. It was only a few days before my 23rd birthday, but instead of looking forward to it, I just wanted to crawl into a hole. I felt like no one in the world understood what it was like to deal with the reality of IBS, how difficult ordinary living had become.

My parents had booked an appointment for me with the local doctor, a nice man who listened carefully to my tale of woe. He was sympathetic and agreed that I should see a gastroenterologist as the symptoms were now interfering with my ability to earn a living.

I also had a blood test at the doctor's office. It was the morning of my birthday and the nurse taking my blood wished me many happy returns. A few days later, the doctor called me to say that I had a low white blood cell count, or "neutropenia." He wasn't sure what that meant in relation to my symptoms, but for the first time in a long time I thought there might actually be something wrong with me that could be treated.

I would go to the doctor, he would give me a bottle of white blood cells to drink, I would drink them and all would be well. Or perhaps not. But at least there was a chance that my illness was treatable and I had a doctor who was trying to help.

In the end, the doctor decided that the low white blood cell count meant nothing whatsoever and was probably just an inaccurate result from the lab. I was still going to see the specialist though. There was definitely hope.

At the specialist

About a week later, my faithful dad drove me to the private hospital where I would see the gastroenterologist. It was a private hospital because I was seeing a private specialist. There were, of course, gastroenterologists available on the National Health Service. That is to say there were about three of them in the whole of England and they only saw patients called Bert. (Or, to put it another way, I was very welcome to see an NHS specialist as long as I didn't mind waiting for months. I minded.)

The specialist was a pleasant enough chap. He took a few brief details of my symptoms and complaints, always a fun way to get to know a stranger. I don't think any of us like discussing our personal bowel habits with doctors, but at the time I was too unhappy to really care about embarrassment.

There were no terrible tests. He did have me lie down so that he could insert his finger into my rectum, which was a charming experience, but that was about it. I also had to give a urine sample, and because this was a hospital, and all hospitals are designed to remove every last shred of your personal dignity, there was no lock on the toilet door and the nurse walked in on me with my trousers down.

After the doctor had finished exploring my rectum and I had finished flashing the nurses, the specialist and I sat together in his office.

He told me that I had IBS, that I needed to avoid constipation and that perhaps I could take a laxative. I sat there, a little stunned, and waited for more advice, for some suggestions about drugs or diet, but none came. I started crying. That was all he could come up with? That was the sum total of his knowledge?

I knew I had IBS, I knew that I needed to avoid constipation, and I was already taking laxatives. We were paying him hundreds of pounds for this? And he was a specialist, for goodness' sake. Gastroenterology school, day one: The colon's connected to the stomach. Day two: Constipated people need laxatives. Day three: Right, you're done now, off you go. Oh no, wait, I forgot, here's how to stick your finger up a rectum.

Looking back, I have to say that his understanding of IBS, both from a medical point of view and from a personal point of view, must have been severely limited for him to suggest nothing but laxatives. Perhaps his sympathy for IBS patients had been eroded by seeing so many of them, tearful and pathetic like I was, and being unable—or unwilling—to do anything to help.

Or maybe he believed that IBS was the name for a neurotic, imaginary illness that afflicts weak little girls who obsess over their bowels and cause all their own problems.

He didn't talk to me about diet or food intolerance or any kind of alternative treatment such as hypnotherapy. He didn't discuss any theories for the causes of IBS or explain where my symptoms might have come from.

He didn't mention any organizations that might have offered some support, and he made me feel like I had come to him with a trivial problem that was not worth his attention. Apparently he was waiting for the colon cancers or the rare gut disorders that would make his name. This girl who was just a bit bunged up (and clearly emotionally deranged) was just filling in time.

At the time I was in no state to argue, but if I ever see the man again . . . well, let's just say that I'll give him a nice long lecture about everything I've learned in the meantime, everything that he had apparently failed to pick up during his many years of training and medical practice. You know, stuff like your diet can affect your digestion, really complicated ideas like that. I'd draw him diagrams and everything.

Once the doctor had finished imparting his wisdom, I left the hospital and went back out to the car with my dad, who of course wanted to know what the doctor had said. I told him, "He thinks it's IBS!" and started to cry yet again.

What I think doctors often misunderstand is that a diagnosis of IBS, while possibly a relief for some patients who have been worrying about cancer or horrific gut-rotting diseases, is actually a life sentence for others. For people like me who have had symptoms for years, and who have done a lot of reading about IBS, being told that it's just IBS is absolutely no comfort whatsoever.

You mean it's just a condition that causes me to spend hours doubled over in pain? Oh, it's just an illness that makes me feel like my stomach's going to explode and my intestines are going to splatter their contents all over the living room, well, that's all right then, as long as it's nothing serious, doctor. You're quite right, I'll go away and shut up. Thank you for your time. Would you like to stick your finger up my rectum?

Although the gastroenterologist had said very little to me in his office, he said rather more in a report of my visit that he sent to the local doctor who had referred me. I was given a copy of this report, and it is shown on the following page.

Allow me to comment on a few items in this report.

"Many thanks for referring this 23-year-old magazine editor to me."
A lovely polite start, but it's a shame about the facts. To be editing an entire magazine at the age of 23 would have been pretty darn impressive, and I

Dr X, Consultant Gastroenterologist
Some hospital, someplace

Many thanks for referring this 23-year-old magazine editor to me. Eleven years ago she suffered with gastroenteritis and since then she has had vague abdominal symptoms.

Generally she sufferers with abdominal discomfort associated with constipation. This has become more troublesome recently although the pain is not severe. She occasionally has diarrhea although largely the pain is in the right flank and there is no loss of weight, appetite or vomiting.

There are no nocturnal symptoms and she has very occasional bright red PR bleeding [blood passed through the rectum]. There is no family history of note. She has taken Colofac in the past with reasonable relief of her symptoms.

On examination she looked well, but was tearful. There was no pallor [skin paleness], jaundice, clubbing [an increase in the soft tissue in the fingers or toes] or lymphadenopathy [disease of the lymph nodes]. Examination of her abdomen was normal, in particular there were no masses, organomegaly [abnormal enlargement of organs] or tenderness. Per rectal examination [digital rectal examination] was normal, as was rigid sigmoidoscopy up to 10cm.

Although her symptoms have been going on for quite a while now, it is unlikely that there is any sinister pathology occurring here and largely her symptoms are of irritable bowel syndrome.

The blood tests you carried out, including full blood count, liver function test, thyroid function test and ESR [erythrocyte sedimentation rate, a test of red blood cells] were all normal except for mild neutropenia [low white blood cell count]. She is due to have an ultrasound scan next week which will be useful for reassuring her.

I have explained that her symptoms are of irritable bowel syndrome and that there are no sinister features. It will be important for her to prevent constipation and magnesium hydroxide [milk of magnesia] would probably be the first choice. I would avoid Lactulose, but if a stronger laxative is needed then small doses of Laxoberal would be useful. Obviously, she should continue to take Colofac.

I did not think that putting her through any further investigations would be useful. I have said that if the situation does not improve or there are new symptoms, then I would be happy to see her again.

Yours sincerely,
Dr X

wasn't. I was an editorial assistant, which is an entry-level job in the publishing world, and as junior as you can get without being the Coke machine. A small point, sure, but I think maybe it says something about the doctor's level of interest in my case.

"And since then she has had vague abdominal symptoms . . ."

I have no idea what the doctor meant by "vague" abdominal symptoms. I had constipation, diarrhea and mild to severe stomach pain. What was vague about that, exactly? And if these are vague symptoms then surely a gastrointestinal specialist would spend an entire career listening to such vagueness. I didn't have constipation for 2.4 days and then three diarrhea attacks on Sundays, but then I didn't realize that such precision was required.

"The pain is not severe."

From what I can recall, the reason he said this was because he had asked me to rate, on a scale of one to 10, the pain that I felt on an average day. I think I said that it was around level four. And, you have to agree, four out of 10 is not severe. Eight or nine out of 10 is severe; four or five is moderate.

But that meant I was in moderate pain for most of the time that I was awake. My average day had become an IBS day by default and I was pretty much in pain or discomfort all the time. That's a bit more than "troublesome." Plus, when I had an extreme IBS attack, the pain was more like an eight, and the worst pain I had ever felt in my entire life ever, but either I didn't get that message across or I wasn't asked about the really bad days that had me sweating and shaking and swearing out loud.

"There is no loss of weight, appetite or vomiting . . ."

This was correct on the weight and vomiting points, but not on the question of appetite. I often lost my appetite when I was constipated, as it felt like the last thing I needed was to add food to my bloated digestive system. Indeed, whenever I get starving hungry it's a sure sign that my bowel is behaving itself.

I don't know why we got our wires crossed here. Maybe it was my fault, maybe it was his. It does show you though how easy it is to miscommunicate with your doctor, and how dangerous this could have been if we hadn't been dealing with "just" IBS.

"On examination she looked well, but was tearful."
I looked well. This is one of my major problems. Even when I am in terrible pain I still look well in the sense that I don't turn green and my arms don't fall off. And yeah, I was tearful. That sounds pathetic, doesn't it? Sighing heroines in romance novels are tearful when their steely-eyed lovers abandon them in favor of the chambermaid. I was completely wretched because I felt like I was being tortured from the inside out.

It's an interesting choice of words. He could have said, "She was clearly very upset," or "She broke down and cried in my office," but he didn't. He chose his words carefully, I guess.

"She is due to have an ultrasound scan next week which will be useful for reassuring her."
This, of course, translates as "useful for reassuring her that she does not have cancer or some other proper disease which she is probably imagining upon herself, the poor, panicky, overanxious tiny child."

I wasn't the least bit worried about cancer or any other scarier condition. In fact, I remember being quite hopeful that the doctor would find something wrong with me that was not IBS, anything that he could treat, anything that he could help me with. I had fantasies about having endometriosis or celiac disease, because then someone might actually sit down with me and talk about how they were going to help.

My greatest fear was that the doctor was going to say I had IBS and I had to just learn to live with it. And that, in the end, was exactly what he said.

* * *

The ultrasound scan came next. It wasn't really explained to me what the scan was looking for, but I had a vague notion that it might be fibroids or a tumor the size of a watermelon, something along those lines.

But I wanted to find out what was wrong with me and get it fixed as soon as possible, even if that meant having test after test. In the end, though, the ultrasound was the only follow-up test that I was given. To this day it is the only investigative mainstream medical test I have had for my IBS (apart from the birthday blood test).

The ultrasound was pretty harmless. The only real problem was the fact that, for some reason, you had to drink about two liters of water before you went to the doctor's office. I think it was something to do with the visibility of the bladder on the scan. So, to make a nice change, I was more worried about wetting myself than pooping. It turned out fine, though, and the actual ultrasound just involved me lying down and having a camera placed on my belly as if I was pregnant.

Nothing showed up on the ultrasound, so at least we had ruled out watermelon-sized growths. But I still didn't have my solution, and it seemed painfully obvious now that I did not have one of my fantasy medical disorders. I had my nightmare medical disorder, and I was stuck with it.

Just to say, if there is anyone reading this who actually has endometriosis or celiac disease, please don't think that I am belittling your condition. I certainly don't envy your symptoms, and every long-term illness comes with its own painful set of symptoms and problems. I didn't really want to be diagnosed with anything at all, of course. I wanted to be well, or at the most to have some specific and easily treatable condition that would show up on a scan and come with a handily simple treatment plan. (Celiac disease, as I would discover later, comes with an easy treatment plan, but endometriosis certainly doesn't—a lesson to be careful what you wish for!)

In reality I was just depressed by the fact that no one seemed to have the first idea how to treat me, and no one even seemed to think that I needed that much help. IBS was a bit of a nuisance to everyone else and a gigantic great nightmare to me.

CHAPTER 6

Clinging to My Job

I HAD TWO CHOICES. I COULD GO BACK TO WORK and tough it out, despite the fact that I'd had no real help from the specialist, or I could quit my job and go to live with my parents.

Both choices seemed pretty gloomy. My parents are lovely people, but if I gave up my job and my flat and took up residence in my childhood home, it would pretty much mean that I had surrendered to my symptoms. What would I do all day? Sit at home and watch TV and think about my useless bowel? What about all the time I had spent working for my degree? But if I went back to work, not only did I have to go back ill, I also had to face my boss and explain why I had taken so much time off work. By that time I had been away for an entire month.

I had given my colleagues very little in the way of explanation as to what was wrong with me. My dad had gone in to see my boss before he drove me home and I think he just said something vague about me not being well and needing some time off. I had definitely not dared to mention anything about my condition to my colleagues, and if I did go back to work, I was presuming that everyone would expect me to go back in a fine state of health, having gotten over my illness in four weeks like normal people do.

During my time off, I had received a letter from my boss who said that things were "very difficult" for them in the office without me because the editorial department I worked in had very few remaining staff. She asked if I could let her know as soon as possible what I was planning to do.

Life was no bed of roses for me either, but I could see where she was coming from. If I had hired someone only to have them disappear four months later I wouldn't be too impressed either, especially when this person seemed to have no explanation for her problems and refused to communicate.

I felt completely trapped between the easy option of quitting my job and lying around, which would leave me with no job, no money and nothing to do all day, or the scary option of returning to work and once again gritting my teeth to make it through the days.

In the end, I decided that I had to go back to work. I don't really know what made up my mind for me, but I remember feeling like I somehow had to cling to the job, and if I could do that, perhaps it would show that I wasn't going to be beaten by the IBS.

So I packed up all my things, my dad drove me back to my flat, and I went back in to work on a Monday morning. It was pretty scary. I had no idea how my colleagues were going to treat me, except that I had the definite impression that I wasn't going to be handed a box of chocolates and told to take it easy.

In the end we dealt with it in the traditional British way—nobody mentioned it. I could tell that things were fairly strained between me and my boss, but we battled on regardless, and after a while things more or less got back to normal between us. As I got through the first week and then the first month of work, I realized that I was, indeed, going to be able to make it.

Perhaps the month off work had been exactly what I needed. It hadn't been lovely and relaxing, but at least it had been a bit of time when I didn't have any responsibilities and didn't have to do the washing up. And I really was determined to keep my job and independence, whatever the state of my bowels.

* * *

Despite my lack of respect for the gastroenterologist I had seen, I decided to follow his advice and try milk of magnesia. Amazingly enough, it did actually help to a certain extent, and it was quite good at tackling the constipation. It wasn't a wonder cure, though, and the state of my digestion was such that I don't think any one approach would have given me significant relief at that time. That's why it was so disappointing that the only advice I had received was to use laxatives.

But still, anything that would take the edge off the symptoms was welcome and I used the milk of magnesia fairly happily for a while. I still occasionally use it for constipation.

I tried very hard not to take any more sick time to compensate for the four weeks I had taken off already. I did have to take one afternoon off when I was shaking and getting terrible cramps, but apart from that I just turned up at the office and stayed there regardless of how I felt.

I even gave up a lot of my holiday time so that I could repay some of my four-week deficit. As soon as I had dragged myself back to work I had started to feel guilty about all of the time I had taken off sick. I was entitled to twenty days' holiday a year, but I only took thirteen days in my last year with the company. I remember e-mailing my dad very proudly one day when I realized that I had worked eleven weeks in a row without a single day off.

It became almost a badge of honor, as if I was trying to prove my worth. I might be in pain and intestinally challenged, but I turned up to work every single day. My gastroenterologist might think that I was pathetic, but I was going to prove him wrong.

In some ways I think that this absolute refusal to give in went way too far. I had been ill, so I deserved some time off and I shouldn't have felt bad about taking it. I definitely deserved my holiday days. Perhaps my guilt was more about the fact that I still didn't quite believe that having IBS was a good enough reason to feel as sick and defeated as I often did.

This was despite the fact that I was still experiencing some major IBS symptoms. For all my determination, I was still in trouble. I hated being sent on reporting jobs out of the office because it meant that I would have to get up early, which would inevitably disturb my stomach. I'd then have to get through a long day feeling dreadful while pretending to feel fine.

Sometimes I had to get up in the middle of the night (well, about 5:30

a.m., which is the middle of the night to any right-thinking person) to go to conferences. I'd have to stay there overnight, which meant more opportunity for problems:

- What food was I going to eat?
- What if I had to eat with people from the conference?
- What if I had to go out in the evening?
- Would anyone mind if I just hid in the toilet?

Because I worked for a publishing company, my colleagues and I sometimes went to exhibitions to sell our books and magazines, and these involved a whole raft of exciting opportunities for pain. Again, I'd have to get up in the middle of the night, sit on a train for a couple of hours, with or without toilet facilities, and then stand at an exhibition stall all day long trying to look cheerful and welcoming rather than miserable and grim.

During one exhibition, I felt ill and very uncomfortable the whole time. When I finally made it through to the end of the day, I caught a lift back to the office with two of my colleagues and sat in the back of the car quietly crying.

It all felt like pointless heroics. Here I was struggling bravely on, through some really tough times, and for what? What was I going to have at the end of it? Nothing, except whatever I had at the start of it, including the IBS.

Needless to say I was still very unhappy during this time. My life basically consisted of getting up (often in pain), going to work (often in pain), coming home and eating, watching TV and going to bed. And yes, all those things were often done in pain.

I would fight tooth and nail to just make it to the weekend, and then I'd find that I couldn't bring myself to do anything useful, like vacuuming or washing the dishes. I'd do the food shopping because starving was out of the question, but anything else had to wait while I did things that I actually enjoyed.

Why? Because I had to get *some* pleasure out of life, I had to have at least a couple of days a week when I could get to the end of the day and think, *Well, that wasn't too traumatic. Wouldn't mind doing that again.*

And it wasn't like I was yachting or hanging out at the Ritz, or even hanging out with my friends; I didn't have the strength for that anyway. It was just the tiny, everyday pleasures like reading a book or playing on my computer. I was desperately seeking something, anything, to let my heart and soul know that my life was not going to be entirely composed of suffering and struggling and lurching from one painful episode to the next.

Even a trip to Legoland turned into an endurance test. I went to organize a competition for the readers of one of our magazines and spent the day being shown around the model villages and children's rides, watching everyone have enormous amounts of fun in the summer sunshine while my stomach felt like it had committed suicide several weeks earlier and was now rotting my body from the inside.

The boss of Legoland had sent a nice lady to show me round, but I couldn't summon up the energy or the will to keep up my side of the conversation. She probably thought I was incredibly rude, but I was exhausted, and it didn't seem to matter one way or the other whether I could make small talk about the weather and the rides. I couldn't really have cared less.

Letters home

My parents had been understandably worried about my return to work, and I had agreed to e-mail them once a week to let them know that I was okay, or if not okay then at least not crying in a corner. Some of these weekly e-mails still survive, buried in the depths of my computer, and as I look through them now I can feel once more how battered I felt back then, and how useless these weekly messages must have been for reassuring my poor parents.

One of the e-mails reads, almost in its entirety:

> Still alive, had major bout yesterday with bad pain and sweating/shaking for a couple of hours, this is what I am doing. Otherwise fine . . .

I'm sure that put my parents' minds at rest.

Here's another:

> I am OK, although tum was a bit bad over the weekend, hence a bit of silence. Is OK now, as OK as it gets, but I was pretty miserable about it. It is like I have a little pool of miserableness that I get stuck in when the IBS comes back, because it's been going on for so long.
>
> If it was anything else I would just go, "Ooh, that's a bit annoying," and watch telly, but stomach pain really gets me down now. Knowing that it's always there, and that even on the good days it feels weird (I had a lovely spasm at work today). That all said, I am feeling better now, and I am trying to make myself believe that the fact that it went on for four days rather than four weeks is an improvement.

One of the interesting things about this e-mail is my use of the word "tum." I remember my dad e-mailing me at about this time and asking me how my "tum" was doing. I read the e-mail and sat there, stewing in a pool of resentment for half an hour, just because I thought that "tum" was a ridiculously cute and fluffy word for the evils of IBS. This one word showed that my dad had no conception of the pain that I was in.

My years of pain had caused me to build up a whole tank of this kind of bile. Some poor unwitting soul would come along and prod me with a slightly inappropriate comment or a mildly insensitive response and I would feel like emptying the entire tank over their head.

My dad, of course, did not deserve to have a tank of bile poured over him, but I needed an outlet for my feelings. I couldn't get angry at my gut, so I got angry at everyone around me.

Some of this sounds very melodramatic, but the trouble is that when I got very low and hopeless I started *feeling* melodramatic, as if every tiny problem was 110 feet tall. When life is going well I have a sense of perspective, but at this time everything around me was viewed through a filter of pain.

In one e-mail I was apparently having a good few weeks for a change, and I said, "I'm a bit bored at the moment, which is always a good sign." It was a good sign because I was never bored when I was sick, as dealing with the symptoms was an activity in itself. It was only when the symptoms abated for a few weeks at a time that I would look around and notice the rest of the world.

Another e-mail said:

> Hi—just wanted to say hi again and sorry again. Really don't mean to worry parents, and then when I do worry parents I worry about worrying parents, so it is a big vicious circle. I know I acted like a miserable git on Saturday, but that is just how it feels sometimes. I am really going to try and get over myself. Don't really like talking about it very much, and I know that makes it worse for you guys, so I will try and keep up e-mail contact as that is easier.
>
> I am going to call the doctor next week, and Ed as well as he is a good cheery-up type person. Am feeling fine today as regards IBS, not perfect, but it is so difficult to live with this all the time.
>
> I think the reason why I don't want to talk to my friends and didn't talk Saturday is that if I had talked and acted "normal" it feels like I'm just pretending that everything is fine.
>
> Basically what I mean is that it is very easy to believe that other people do not understand what it is like and I'll end up sitting there having a normal conversation while I can feel my intestine having a spasm, and I'm supposed to pretend that nothing is happening. I've done that so often in the past. I've got this whole list of things that I acted my way through while feeling bad: exams, interviews, loads of holidays, weekends away, day trips, days at work, 21st birthday.
>
> I think I've just run out of strength a bit at the moment to carry on doing that and have descended into feeling sorry for myself and deciding that I shouldn't have to pretend. My solution to that is not to speak to anyone.
>
> I know it's difficult to imagine what it's like for an IBS person. It's just the first thing I think about, so often. For example, Dad

asked me whether there were any more day trips to London coming up. For anyone else, this would be an exciting thing. But the first thing I think of when I hear "day trip" is pain. Those two days I had in London last time were bad IBS days and I had to stand there with a smile on my face all day and just get through it. My digestive system is so sensitive that I have to constantly think about the consequences of my actions or I'll get into trouble again.

I hope that this has maybe explained a few things. I promise to sort myself out. I am very sorry for making you feel bad, but I think my brain figured it deserved to feel sorry for itself for a while.

Please try not to worry too much, as I'm going to be OK. I don't want to be the reason you're unhappy—that's horrible. But I also have to be able to tell you what's going on, and not pretend.

I was not a happy bunny.

CHAPTER 7

Hypnotherapy, Gluten, Fiber and Magnesium

I DECIDED THAT I HAD TO TRY SOMETHING DIFFERENT in order to stay afloat. I looked through the Yellow Pages for a therapist or alternative medicine practitioner who might be able to help, and I came across an ad for hypnotherapy.

From the books I had read I knew that hypnotherapy was one of the more commonly used therapies for IBS, and there certainly didn't seem to be any danger of doing more harm than good. It wasn't as if I was going to be swallowing a load of unidentified pills or getting needles stuck in my arm; I was just going to be a bit sleepy.

The only thing that I had against hypnotherapy was the fact that it seemed to be treating my mind instead of my body. I now know that this isn't true. Just because hypnotherapy works for some IBS sufferers does not mean to say that their problems are psychological. Hypnotherapy is so powerful that it can even be used instead of anesthesia to dull the pain of operations.

Despite my slight reservations about the treatment, I decided to go ahead, partly because I needed something to cling to and partly because the therapist lived very conveniently halfway between my flat and my office, so I could visit him on the way home from work.

I called the therapist up and he invited me to his home office for a free initial consultation. During this consultation I had to fill in a questionnaire to explain the symptoms that were troubling me. The questionnaire in itself almost made me feel better, as it covered all kinds of different conditions and life situations that might be bothering a person, everything from anxiety and depression to homosexuality and divorce. I hardly ticked any of the boxes and felt almost normal. My bowel was my only problem.

The therapist then asked me to sum up, in one or two words, what I would most wish for in the world as a result of his treatment. I said, "freedom." That sounds a bit dramatic, but I was told that it was actually a very common thing for IBS sufferers to say. Even if you try to take your mind off IBS you are constantly forced to think about it, and not just because you are in crippling pain or can't get out of the bathroom.

If you are going out to eat or going on a trip or cooking a meal, you have to think about it. If you are planning to change jobs or move house, you have to think about it. If you have to get up at a different time in the morning or go to bed at a different time at night, you have to think about it.

Sufferers often find that they need strict morning routines to minimize the pain. They might have to get up at 6 a.m. to be on time for their 9 a.m. jobs, or they might need to have coffee an hour before they leave the house or eat fiber every time they have an evening meal.

All of this left me with a very rigid life that didn't allow for any deviations. If I changed any one thing without warning, I would pay for it later. I needed to be free from this rigidity and from the constant threat of symptoms; it was suffocating.

The therapist explained to me how the hypno would work. I felt comfortable with the guy and it all sounded quite hopeful, so I booked some sessions. Plus he had a very nice cat.

The hypnotherapy itself was rather nice. The therapist would gently coax me into a kind of hyperrelaxed state, with some calm music playing in the background. Then he would ask me to visualize things such as a healthy stomach and a working digestive system or ask me to hold my hand over my stomach and feel a healing warmth flow from my hand into my gut.

I never really felt like I was hypnotized. It was more like being very, very relaxed. It's a million miles from stage hypnosis though, just in case you're wondering. I was still aware of my surroundings and still in control of my actions. At no time did I bark like a dog.

Although hypnotherapy does work well for some people, it didn't really do that much for me, although it was certainly very relaxing. My symptoms continued to vary from week to week, without much appreciable improvement.

Still, I do think that it probably helped me from an emotional point of view, because it was lovely just to have someone ask me how I was feeling every week. After all, no one at work ever asked me that, because they didn't know that I was suffering. It was good to be able to say how I felt.

This is in fact one of the concrete benefits of alternative or complementary therapies. While there's no doubt that some of them are built on very questionable science (or no science at all), one huge advantage of almost all of them is that you get a significant period of time sitting quietly in a room with someone who listens to you, sympathizes and then sets out a comprehensive plan of treatment.

I don't know about you, but I have never received this kind of treatment from a mainstream doctor. Now, I know they're busy, I know they're stressed and I know IBS isn't easy to treat. But a good bedside manner is far more important than many doctors seem to think, and good listening skills and a simple belief that a patient's symptoms are genuinely painful can work wonders.

There is a basic human need to have our pain acknowledged. If you want to test this theory, try this out on a nearby child: The next time the little tyke falls over and says, "It really hurts!" tell them that of course it doesn't hurt, and see what happens.

If just one doctor had sincerely told me that IBS was a devil to live with and I was coping rather well, I would have offered to have his babies.

Anyway, the hypnotherapy hadn't made much difference, but it was a start. I had spent some time with a very kind man who listened to me, believed me when I said I was hurting and let me stroke his cat.

Just the knowledge that I was actively trying to get rid of my symptoms was comforting. I hadn't yet given up hope.

Going gluten-free

Following the hypnotherapy failure, I decided to try altering my diet. I had read various versions of suggested diets for IBS sufferers, some conflicting, some downright ridiculous, but one suggestion that kept coming up was to cut out gluten.

Gluten is a protein that's found in wheat, barley and rye, and it's often found on the lists of top-10 foods that can cause gut problems. It's also the culprit for celiac disease sufferers, and some parents use gluten-free diets for their autistic children as well. There's clearly something about the stuff that causes problems in sensitive people and I was nothing if not sensitive.

To help me with the diet, I arranged a phone consultation with a nutritionist. She advised a pretty radical change in diet that included some things that were really not going to happen, such as changing almost all of my food habits and staple meals and basically switching to someone else's diet overnight.

IBS patients are often so exhausted by their symptoms that they don't have the strength to follow even the most well-intentioned advice. To me, an entirely new diet was about as obtainable as an entirely new gut.

"All you have to do, person who's been in pain for 12 years and is clinging to life by the fingernails, is change every single aspect of your diet and lifestyle and you'll feel so much better."

"But I don't have the energy of half a dead firefly, how am I going to do that?"

"I really have no idea, but eat more anchovies."

Actually that's unfair to the nutritionist, who was very nice and only trying to help. I have no idea whether her suggestions would have helped me or not, but I did know that in my current state of decrepitude there was no way I could manage to change my habits so exhaustively.

After all, a massive change in diet can be almost impossible to achieve even if you're perfectly healthy. We build up eating habits over years and years, and breaking those habits takes a considerable amount of effort and willpower. Anyone who has tried to lose weight will know how easy it is in theory and how difficult in practice.

However, the nutritionist did say that going gluten-free could well be a good start, if not the whole solution. This seemed like one practical, not completely daunting thing that I could do. Therefore, I decided that cutting out gluten was the best way to go.

Unfortunately, it wasn't quite as simple as I'd hoped. If you've never tried not eating gluten then you won't know that it's not easy. (That's the worst sentence in the world, I do apologize.)

What I mean is that gluten gets in everything; it's not just a case of swearing off the doughnuts. You have to read the label of every single packet in the supermarkets, constantly on alert for little particles of the stuff.

So not only do you have to cut out all the obvious foods, like bread, pasta, cakes and biscuits, but also a wide range of not-so-obvious foods, and even some entirely ridiculous where-in-the-heck-is-the-gluten-in-that foods. Gluten is used as filler in all sorts of things, from sausages to soup, and the only way to find it is to check the labels religiously. Even then the gluten sometimes remains hidden under vague terms like "starch."

(Reading the labels on foods is an education in itself. I couldn't help wondering if all of these unidentifiable ingredients that I was eating might have something to do with the sorry state of my digestion. I mean, a potato is a potato, but what the hell is monosodium glutamate anyway?)

Still, if I had to scrupulously read labels to embark on my gluten-free adventure, then that's what I would do. One development that made things easier was that supermarkets began to add allergy advice labels to everything they sold. I think this was in response to the peanut situation, where allergy sufferers could literally drop down dead if they ate a tiny amount of peanut, but it was also a great help for people like me because gluten was one of the ingredients identified on the labels.

I also went to a health food shop and bought some gluten-free bread, pasta and biscuits. I discovered fairly quickly that while gluten-free foods have no gluten in them, they often have no taste in them either, nor any resemblance to the gluten-filled version of whatever they are pretending to be.

Bread in particular is an umbrella term for all kinds of stuff in the gluten-free world, from crumbly cake-type concoctions to a moist and squidgy swamp loaf. It's very expensive and the slices are very small, so you now have four sandwiches to a lunch where before you had two, and even the best gluten-free breads are still prone to crumbling and having their corners fall off.

On the other hand, gluten-free pasta tastes almost exactly like pasta, which is all I was asking from the stuff. The biscuits were pretty nice too, so it wasn't all bad.

My nutritionist's company had published a book about IBS, *No More IBS!* by Maryon Stewart and Dr. Alan Stewart, and this provided some useful guidance about what I was supposed to be eating. The book also explained how to follow a full-on exclusion diet. This involves excluding different groups of foods in different weeks, for a period of ten weeks, and seeing how each food group affected your symptoms.

So for example, during one week you stop eating citrus fruit; during another, you exclude gluten; and in another, you stop eating dairy (IBS sufferers often react to any one or all of these foods). This seemed like a very sensible and thorough approach, but the required amount of organization and dedication was simply beyond me.

I look at my copy of *No More IBS!* now and remember how much I needed something to believe in. I have even highlighted parts of the book that say the dietary changes may take some weeks to take effect. I remember trying very hard to convince myself that I would definitely feel better very soon, and if I could just hold on for a little bit longer the pain would be over.

Thankfully, I found that after a few weeks on the new gluten-free diet, I did indeed feel noticeably better. I wasn't cured by any means, but I had fewer stomachaches and I felt a bit more positive about life. A little hope had finally been rewarded with some genuine results, and this looked promising.

Fiber and magnesium

The nutritionist also suggested that I try taking fiber supplements and magnesium tablets: fiber because it can help with the whole spectrum of IBS symptoms, and magnesium tablets because they can work as a mild laxative and help relieve the constipation.

I'd tried fiber before in the shape of the Fybogel that my university doctor had given me. Like most things, it didn't seem to do much good, although it was difficult to tell because of the day-to-day fluctuations of IBS. I didn't really want to go back to the Fybogel though, so I decided to choose a different kind of fiber.

This was a major decision in itself. There are about six squillion different types of fiber and seven squillion different formulations: with sugar, without sugar, in powder form or tablet form, in orange flavor, lemon flavor, no flavor, etc.

For some reason that now escapes me, I decided to try two types at once —Normacol (sterculia fiber) and Celevac (methylcellulose). I really would not recommend this, because how can you tell which fiber is working (if it is working)? Also, what if one agrees with you and one doesn't and you've just ruled them both out unilaterally? It really was rather hare-brained.

On the other hand, it was rather brilliant, because for whatever reason the combination of fibers worked very well for me, and chipped away a little more at the IBS monster.

Magnesium was something that I'd never tried before, at least not in tablet form. My gastro specialist had advised me to take magnesium hydroxide, or milk of magnesia to us lay people, and I'd tried that for a while. It did seem to help with the constipation, but it hadn't been a cure by itself.

However, the nutritionist wasn't suggesting that I take milk of magnesia; she was suggesting plain old magnesium tablets. Magnesium in many different forms has a mild laxative effect, and calcium tablets have the opposite effect. I would later find out that there are hundreds, if not thousands, of IBS sufferers who use magnesium or calcium tablets for their IBS symptoms, and that these minerals are two very famous treatments within online IBS communities.

I bought some magnesium citrate tablets to add to my regimen. I also bought some tablets that contained both calcium citrate and magnesium citrate, and some vitamin D capsules as well. The calcium and vitamin D were more for my dodgy back than for the IBS, but I started taking them all at around the same time. Again, this was not the brightest way of doing things, but by sheer luck I had hit on another positive combination and my symptoms eased even further.

In fact, much to my immense relief, the combination of all of these things together seemed to hit a magic button and I had several days of feeling very well. Then several weeks. Then several months. Once I had passed two whole months, I was incredulous but fantastically relieved, as I had never had two months off from my symptoms before in the entire history of my IBS.

This was something to get excited about. I was 24 by this point, and I'd had IBS for well over a decade. In all of that time I had never experienced relief like this.

And not only was I feeling very well in general, with no pain or discomfort or bloating, but I was also producing the most spectacularly well-formed bowel movements in the whole long history of the world. These were Olympian, Ivy League bowel movements, so perfect in size and shape that had you clapped eyes on one of them, you would surely have said, "Goodness me, that is the finest bowel movement I have ever seen in my whole life. Very well done, Miss Lee."

There, you really wanted to know that didn't you? You've been waiting for that one, right? I bet you only bought this book to get intimate descriptions of my poop. I aim to please. Shall I draw you a little picture? Maybe later.

IBS is my default position

Despite the fact that I was doing so well on my new regimen, I had noticed a rather unfortunate side effect of fighting the IBS monster for so long: I was now terrified of it coming back, and for good reason.

It had always, always come back before, like one of those horror movie monsters that goes "Aarrrggh" when it is shot and stabbed and burned and then comes back to life three minutes later when the teenager going to the prom finds the old abandoned cemetery and decides that the best thing to do is dance around naked while vomiting on the gravestones. It was almost exactly like that.

This was a big issue for me. On the one hand, I had stumbled across the first real hope that I could subdue the IBS symptoms to almost nothing. On the other hand, I had come to this situation so haphazardly that I didn't really know why it was working or whether it would stop at any moment. I didn't even know if the fiber and the magnesium and the lack of gluten were the secrets to my relief. Maybe it was something completely random, like the fact that I'd stopped eating oranges.

IBS is such an inexplicable disorder anyway, with attacks often coming out of thin air and then disappearing just as mysteriously, that it seemed ridiculous to think that I had finally fallen upon a solution. It is very difficult to really relax and enjoy life when you are constantly wondering whether today will be the day when your symptoms return. IBS is not cured; it is managed.

I also had to remind myself that even healthy people get bowel problems occasionally. Human beings are not perfect machines, and it is normal to suffer from diarrhea or constipation from time to time. It's almost impossible for an IBS sufferer to distinguish between normal fluctuations and IBS symptoms, but I tried to make sure that my expectations of my digestive system were not wildly unrealistic.

This means that I had to be careful when analyzing poop. You know what I mean by "analyzing poop," right? (If you don't know what that means then I don't think you have IBS. Stop reading this book immediately, you rogue healthy person.)

Analyzing poop, just in case you've never done this (and if you haven't, I highly recommend it as a pleasant way to spend an afternoon) simply involves having a poop and then making a number of assumptions about your general state of health based on the output of your intestines.

In some ways this is a legitimate thing to do, because if your poop is very loose or very hard then that means something is going wrong somewhere. The problem is that there are a whole range of poops between loose and hard that are considered normal. Non-sufferers probably take no notice of the format of their bowel movements, but IBS sufferers often find themselves looking to their stools as an indication of their level of health.

It strikes me that IBS and other bowel conditions are quite special in this respect, and it's no wonder that we sometimes become rather fixated on our movements. I mean, our particular illness provides us with a regular (or irregular) update on the condition of our insides in handy poop form. You don't get that with diabetes.

When the magnesium and fiber combination kicked in, my poops became super-humanly perfect, but occasionally I would still have a less-than-perfect poop and I would see that as an indication that things might be going wrong again. In reality, it usually meant nothing of the sort, but it was difficult not to get scared.

I did know that the most important thing was whether I was pain-free and comfortable, and as long as my movements weren't ridiculously strange there was nothing to worry about. But I still found myself imbued with a sense of quiet pride on the days when my poops were perfect, and a mild sense of impending doom when they weren't.

So my life was much improved in terms of my health, but nothing much else had changed. I didn't dare start traveling or drinking or staying over at friends' houses because I was so sure this would upset the delicate balance I had achieved. My diet was healthy but repetitive, and I was still limited to a basic kind of life.

Now, I didn't have many complaints about that, as I had never been the type of person who wants to backpack around Thailand or drink until four in the morning. But I did want to see the future. Had I really found my cure?

CHAPTER 8

Coming Out of the IBS Closet

IT WAS AROUND THIS TIME THAT I STARTED TO TELL a few more people that I had irritable bowel syndrome, slowly making my way out of the IBS closet. Up until this point the only people I had told were my parents (and through them my brother) and my friend at university who had wanted to go InterRailing around Europe.

My parents had been extremely supportive and helpful, and my friend had been as sympathetic as he could be. He didn't really have a concept of the impact that IBS can have, mostly because I hadn't been able to explain it to him properly, but at least he had accepted me and my condition and been kind about it.

I didn't want to come out as an IBS sufferer at work because I was just too embarrassed. My colleagues were nice and friendly, but the thought of going into work one day and striking up a jolly conversation about my bowel habits just seemed mortifying beyond belief.

My head would tell me that there was no reason to be embarrassed: I hadn't done anything wrong, I wasn't torturing small furry animals to death in the basement, and there was absolutely no reason to feel ashamed. But it wasn't enough to overcome the taboo on any kind of talk about bowels.

Not only was the IBS embarrassing, it also made me vulnerable. If you reveal anything personal or intimate or socially unacceptable about yourself, you are immediately giving people the power to mock you or judge you, just because they feel like it. You have to trust people to be mature and not childish, kind instead of cruel, open-minded rather than smugly judgmental.

To this day I don't really know what my colleagues thought was wrong with me. I had taken a whole month off work, so they obviously knew that something was awry. But I had never handed in the doctor's note that had "irritable bowel syndrome" printed on it, and I didn't even say I had a gut problem. I just didn't say much of anything and tried to pretend I was healthy. It's very easy to look back now and think that I should have just gathered my courage, sat everyone down and said, "This is how it is, please cut me some slack." At the time it seemed impossible.

I did start telling some of my friends though, and this wasn't as horrific as I had feared. Nobody laughed at me, nobody made fun of me, and it did feel good to let people know what was going on rather than trying to hide it all the time.

It also made it much easier to cope with restaurant outings or barbecues, as I could now legitimately turn down gluten-filled foods without looking anorexic or ungrateful. My lovely friends would even buy what they called "Sophie-friendly" food to make sure I had something to eat, bless their hearts. There were a number of occasions when I turned up somewhere and found that the hosts had made a special effort to make sure I had a gluten-free version of whatever everyone else was eating.

However, there was something bothering me about a few of the reactions I'd received, and it was the same problem I'd had with my gastro specialist and indeed all the doctors I had spoken to. There seemed to be a very large gap between some people's perceptions of the seriousness of IBS and my own experiences.

Non-sufferers seemed to think that IBS was a mild condition that caused diarrhea and a bit of pain, but nothing that you couldn't cope with easily as long as you watched your diet or took some pills.

And even though I was actually controlling the IBS at the time with diet and pills, it never felt remotely easy. The years of suffering I had gone through meant that I saw IBS as a mountain where non-sufferers saw a molehill. If there's one thing in life guaranteed to get my goat (and it takes a lot to get my goat, he's tethered very carefully to a hippo) it's people assuming that IBS is a minor inconvenience.

There are even people who refuse to believe that IBS exists, and who therefore try to tell you that your symptoms are perfectly normal aspects of human existence because we all have diarrhea from time to time and you're just exaggerating. These IBS deniers belong to a happy little band of people who seem to think that any medical condition that has not been completely explained and dissected by medical science is baloney and not to be indulged.

Even the people who accepted that there was something wrong with me were baffled by my odd behavior and feeble explanations. Before I had found my new magic treatment regimen, I'd had a friend come to stay with me for a week. I had ended up crying in front of him one night because it felt like he didn't understand what it was like to spend your life in pain.

He didn't understand why I acted weird about only having one bathroom (and asked him to say when he might be in it); he didn't understand why I wanted to be left alone sometimes; and he didn't understand why I ended up crying when I tried to explain why I was upset. It felt like I was on a different planet.

Another friend said, "Don't let it rule your life." That one really got to me. The IBS *completely* ruled my life, from top to bottom. It was stronger than me, bigger than me, it was eating me alive—and I was supposed to just resist? "Yes, but don't *let* the nasty lion eat you, Mr. Wildebeest. Show some guts."

I began to feel a sense of failure because I wasn't living up to other people's expectations of how I should be coping with my illness. Everyone from my friends to my gastro specialist seemed to expect me to muddle through regardless, and they didn't seem to think this was too much to ask.

I was used to meeting people's expectations. I was a well-behaved girl who got good grades at school and did her homework. I wasn't used to feeling like people were disappointed in me or thought that I should pull my socks up and improve.

At the same time I felt angry that people's expectations suddenly seemed to have skyrocketed. Before I had developed IBS, the people in my life expected me to behave and work hard and pass exams and go to university and get a job. I did all of these things, and I had to work very hard sometimes, but the goals were never beyond my grasp, and they were things that I expected of myself as well.

But now I was expected to pass the IBS equivalent of a PhD in nuclear physics, and everyone was staring at me with concerned, puzzled looks on their faces, saying, "We don't understand, Miss Lee, what part of advanced theoretical proton fission seems to be giving you the trouble?"

What I really wanted from someone was a simple acknowledgment that irritable bowel syndrome is a right bugger to cope with. I wanted someone to be really, properly shocked when they heard that I had IBS so I could feel like it was okay to be so worn down and exhausted.

My fantasy conversation with a non-sufferer would go a little something like this:

Me: I've been feeling quite ill lately.

Non-sufferer: Oh, I'm sorry to hear that. What seems to be the trouble?

Me: I have irritable bowel syndrome.

Non-sufferer: Oh, my goodness gracious, irritable bowel syndrome! That's so *awful,* what a terrible burden! I am deeply sorry and distressed to hear you are dealing with such a pernicious and difficult condition. Please accept my heartfelt sympathy on behalf of myself and my many friends and relations.

Me: Oh, thank you, I appreciate that.

Non-sufferer: Although I know that IBS is very difficult to live with, I am very ignorant about the causes of the condition and its treatments. Indeed, I have only read a few articles about it in magazines, which means that I really know next to nothing and I clearly need to be educated. Could you tell me more so I might learn?

Me: Certainly [explains more about IBS].

Non-sufferer: Well, that is all exceedingly interesting, I am so glad you have told me more. I would also like to mention that I am not in the least bit embarrassed about discussing this, as going to the bathroom is a natural bodily function and I am over the age of two. Please could you describe your symptoms in great detail?

Me: [Describes symptoms in great detail.]

Non-sufferer: That really does sound terrible. I am so sorry you have to put up with this. You must always let me know if I can help in any way, and if I say anything cretinous you must slice off my nose with a bread knife.

No one ever says that, though.

Now, I do realize that in many respects I'm asking for way too much from people. There's no excuse for rudeness and treating me like a leper because my bowels have gone bananas, but it's very difficult for people without IBS to know exactly what it entails. The same applies to any other medical problem.

For example, if you met someone tomorrow and they told you that they suffered from cluster headaches, what would you say? "Oh, sorry about that," maybe, or "Oh dear, that's a pity. Would you like a cup of tea?" You probably don't know anything about cluster headaches, so you assume they're some form of headache-type condition, and they probably cause a bit of pain, and you should act sympathetic and then start talking about the weather. The cluster headache sufferer would then be entitled to spontaneously combust all over your jumper.

Cluster headaches are also known as suicide headaches, and they are one of the most painful medical conditions on the planet. The pain is described by some sufferers as like having a red-hot poker in your eye. Attacks can go on for hours.

Once you've learned what cluster headaches are, you'll treat any sufferers you meet with respect. However, ignorance of a medical problem is, much as I hate to admit it, an excuse for a certain amount of insensitivity.

Still, that doesn't change the fact that the gap between my experience of IBS and other people's perceptions only served to make me feel more alone and puny and add to my distress.

I partly blame the name. If you've got an irritable cough it doesn't mean that you're in pain for months on end, so an irritable bowel can't be that bad, can it? It just doesn't sound like a serious condition. (My suggestions for a replacement name include Machete Shreds the Gut Syndrome and Dear God Just Shoot Me Now Bowel.)

Bowels are very funny

I wasn't just dealing with reactions from my friends and family. As someone who was now hypersensitive about her bowels I started to notice bathroom humor in all kinds of TV shows and films. Needless to say, I very rarely found it funny.

There's an episode of *Friends* where Ross has a guilty secret: he had food poisoning at Disneyworld and messed his pants. During the course of the show the writers get at least three huge laughs from this fact. Now, I love *Friends*. It's one of my favorite shows of all time, but even in the fluffy, good-hearted world of Ross and Rachel, I'm a joke.

There are jokes about bowels in plenty of films too. *Along Came Polly* gave Ben Stiller IBS just to poke fun at him. I can't bring myself to watch it because I know I'll end up depressed. Imagine going to the movie theater and sitting there surrounded by people who are laughing at the one thing in your life that makes you completely, unutterably miserable.

But isn't it, like, hilarious if you have to use the bathroom and there's *totally* no paper, can you imagine the *mess*? Yes I can, actually. Thanks for asking.

Then there's the *Sex and the City* movie. The girls go on holiday to Mexico and Charlotte messes her pants; so far so ordinary. But the incident is presented as being not only extraordinarily funny, but so out-and-out pant-wettingly hilarious that it lifts Carrie out of an enormous depression that nothing else could touch.

You might tell me to lighten up, that it's just a comedy, and toilet humor is just harmless fun. But these jokes condemn anyone with a bowel problem to a lifetime of laughter—other people's. There's a huge difference between laughing at a generic bottom joke and making fun of someone's suffering.

If we're taught that diarrhea is funny, what the hell are we supposed to do when we find ourselves going to the bathroom ten times a day and pooping our pants in the greengrocer's? Laugh at ourselves, I suppose, but it's not that simple.

What this situation does is heap embarrassment on people who are struggling quite enough already. IBS patients often put up with symptoms for years before seeing a doctor because they are so embarrassed and humiliated by their symptoms and so terrified of the reactions of others. This appalling state of affairs only exists because of these childish attitudes and useless taboos.

And it's not just IBS patients who suffer in silence: it's people with Crohn's disease, with celiac disease, with colitis, with hemorrhoids, with rectal prolapses and colostomy bags and bowel cancer. Isn't digestion *funny*?

And it's all so incredibly unfair. Imagine a scene where Charlotte is struggling to breathe because of asthma and the other girls are sat around guffawing at her suffering. There is no way in the world that anyone would think that was funny, and if you wrote that scene it would portray the laughing girls as unbelievably cruel and unfeeling. So why is it okay to show people laughing at pain if the pain is located in your gut?

And yet, having said all that, you may have noticed that I do occasionally joke about my condition. That is very different from other people making fun of my IBS, which is strictly forbidden and gives me the immediate right to decapitate you. (I once described to someone how I had been crying because of the pain and my listener actually laughed. Why? He thought I was making a joke about a mild stomach complaint causing intense pain, which clearly would never happen.)

But I'm allowed to make fun of it. My IBS is an extremely powerful force in my life, and if I can mock it and expose it for the ridiculous, mysterious, unsatisfactorily inexplicable condition that it is, maybe that will take away some of its power. It does work, to an extent. Occasionally I can see the funny side of needing a good half an hour in which to poop and even then not doing it properly. (Are you laughing at the back there? Cut it out.)

Mostly though I take my IBS very, very seriously, and I resent anyone who thinks they're entitled to laugh at me just because my illness happens to involve my bowel. I deserve as much respect and empathy as anyone else who is ill, and to rob me of that respect because of something that is out of my control is cruel and unusual punishment.

Reactions out of time

I was also beginning to find that some people talked to me as if I had only just developed symptoms and didn't know the first thing about IBS. They gave advice that might have been helpful to a person who had had symptoms for a week but was useless for someone who had now been suffering for over a decade.

IBS sufferers often get advised by friends and family to go to the doctor or stop worrying, but people will also suggest trying peppermint oil, or laxatives, or fiber supplements, or whatever else they have just read about in their newspaper.

Now, if you've just found out that you have IBS, then these may be moderately useful suggestions. But by that time I'd had IBS for twelve years. What did everyone think I'd been doing all this time, learning to spell it?

The list of daft comments that I heard about IBS grew and grew. Whenever I read an article on IBS or the story of a fellow sufferer on the Internet, I found another ridiculous remark that showed a complete misunderstanding of the whole basis of IBS.

Even the people who were supposed to be helping us, the doctors and nurses and healthcare professionals, often treated us as if we were whining wimps. Fellow sufferers seemed to spend as much time fighting ignorance and intolerance as they did fighting their disease.

TOP-10 STUPID THINGS SAID TO IBS SUFFERERS, AND THE REASONS WHY THEY'RE SO DUMB

1. It is caused by something you are eating so you should avoid that food to get better.

This appears to be perfectly logical. If you are doing something that hurts you, such as ramming a skewer through your foot, you are best advised to stop that activity.

However, the trouble with this particular piece of logic is that it assumes three things. First, that food is the cause of all IBS symptoms; second, that you know exactly what food is causing the trouble; and third, that you can easily eliminate that food without causing more problems. None of these things are true.

This particular quote does make me angry because it also assumes that you, the IBS sufferer, are such a complete and total moron that you don't even have the mental capacity to stop eating, say, oranges, even when every time you eat an orange you get sick. It is not that simple.

2. You should go to the toilet before we leave so we don't have to stop on the way.

This one shows that the speaker has not really grasped the phrase "irritable bowel." It is not a bowel that malfunctions but then pulls itself together when we need to go and visit Great Aunt Maud. Nor is it a bowel that can be relieved and then put back to sleep.

If I am going to have diarrhea in the car then that is where I am going to have diarrhea, whether I have been to the bathroom or not.

3. Why don't you just try this lovely bread/pizza/chili? A little bit won't hurt you.

A rough translation of this is as follows:

"Why don't you just eat a little of this food that gives you stomach pains that feel like there's a chainsaw-wielding hacksaw-waving madman inside your intestines, I won't be the one who has to deal with it and I'm a generally insensitive oaf."

4. **Oh yes, my mother had IBS, but she took a pill from the health food store/ate some bran/stopped eating oranges and now she's cured. Why don't you do that?**

If your mother took one pill and was cured, she did not have IBS. If I took one pill from the health food store, I might be a little bit healthier, but I would not be cured of IBS.

Furthermore, to assume that what "cured" your mother's IBS will "cure" mine is a little naïve. Does it work that way for any other illness? Do all epilepsy sufferers do the same thing to cure themselves? Do all arthritis patients stop eating oranges and get better?

If one more person tells me how to cure my IBS then I shall stab them.

5. **I had that last weekend.**

You describe your symptoms and someone says, "Oh yes, I had that the other day, but I'm much better now thanks."

No, you had a stomach bug or drank too much. You did not have IBS. That's like saying you have clinical depression when you've been feeling a bit gloomy for three minutes. Have you had a stomachache for twenty years? No? Well, be quiet then.

6. **Why don't you go to the doctor?**

I love this one. It's partly the idea that, again, the IBS sufferer is so brain-addled that the very idea of going to the doctor has not occurred to them—they tried asking for advice from the paperboy, but he really wasn't that much help.

And I also love the complete naïveté of the person who thinks that doctors cure everything. I suppose it's usually strappingly healthy people who say this, people who go to the doctor once every ten years for some minor complaint, get some tablets and get cured. So, naturally, that's how it works for us as well.

Everyone from the arthritis sufferer to the Crohn's disease patient knows that there are many situations where doctors can only help you manage your symptoms. Sometimes they don't even do that.

And when we do go to the doctor, we're often treated pretty badly. I suppose this is partly understandable. If I was a doctor I would want to have as few IBS patients as possible, because we can be very difficult to treat.

However, this does not excuse the fact that IBS patients frequently come out of the doctor's office feeling worse than when they went in. They feel like the doctor belittled their problems, gave them no new advice, or implied that their symptoms were neurosis in disguise. Doctors can be disappointing people.

7. You're only talking about your symptoms to get attention.

To be honest I'd hope that your wife/husband/best friend would never dream of saying this one, but it's certainly something that is said to many suffering IBSers.

And you can see where they're coming from. If I was feeling unwanted and in need of some attention, the first thing I would do is pretend to have a bowel problem. Yes, you lonely people! Say that you're so constipated you haven't pooped for three weeks and you'll get all the attention you want.

8. I know that you have IBS, but if you don't go to this meeting/go on this trip/take this course, you're fired.

Most employers, of course, are not as blunt as this, but that's often what they mean. IBS sufferers often find that they have to take a lot of time off work and they sometimes miss very important meetings or events. It can be almost impossible to travel.

But what are we supposed to do? Turn up to the meeting and sit there in excruciating pain? Turn up and run to the bathroom every five minutes while still in excruciating pain? Turn up to the meeting and crap ourselves to prove we're ill? From what I hear, we often do. You'd be amazed at how much pain and discomfort we can ignore just so we can keep our jobs.

If there was a visible sign on every sufferer to show how much pain we were in, no one would accuse us of malingering.

9. What do you mean you're ill again—I thought you said you were feeling better?

I did say that, but that was last week. This week I feel like death. Next week I may feel like a banana. It varies quite a lot, you know.

You get better after having a cold. If you have IBS you get better periodically and sick periodically, in a lovely little cycle that goes on and on and on.

At first, people are very sorry to hear that you are ill, give you some proper sympathy, and ask if there is anything they can do to help. They ask how you are feeling after a week has passed, and then again after another week. They're still fairly sorry after a month. After six months, they decide that you're a malingerer and should be shot.

And last but not least, the most overused phrase in the IBS universe:

10. It's all in your head.

This is, in my opinion, just about the most unsympathetic response an IBS sufferer can get. How is it helpful? How is it supportive? Are you saying that if I just had the courage, the self-possession, the huge emotional capacity that you yourself possess, I could control my bowels?

Because that's how you control your own bowels, is it not? Every day, through a magnificent feat of mental agility, you direct your digestive system to work smoothly, and if I could just do this too I would be well on the way to good health.

Wait a minute, you say you *don't* control your bowels with your mind? What do you mean you just go to the bathroom when your body tells you to—I thought you had a sophisticated mind-bowel control system going on?

So that's the first thing. Bowels are not controlled by our heads. Yes, if you get nervous then you sometimes need the loo, and yes, there is obviously a mechanism that causes certain emotions to affect the bowel, just as negative emotions and stress can make all kinds of illnesses worse, from asthma to multiple sclerosis.

There is also some research to suggest that IBS is at least partly caused by a complex brain-gut interaction, which leaves IBS sufferers far more sensitive to pain and normal gut contractions than regular people.

But that is not what you are saying, is it? You are saying that my entire IBS experience, for all those years, through good and bad times, has been caused by the fact that I'm neurotic. This is total rubbish.

Not only does this response summarily dismiss all of the evidence for causes such as food intolerance and bacterial overgrowth, it also places all blame for the illness squarely at the door of the IBS sufferer. "It's your fault," they are saying. "Get a grip. Snap out of it."

What a complete pile of unadulterated piffle. If anyone ever tells you that your symptoms are in your head, I want you to demand a 100-page, scientific, peer-reviewed, footnoted paper on why they believe this is true. And then I want you to hit them quite hard with a brick.

Disclaimer

You may be reading this and thinking, *Wow, this girl is angry!* It may even be that you are the friend of an IBS sufferer and you have said some of the things listed above, thinking that they were perfectly rational and helpful remarks.

At the time, with the knowledge you had then, they probably seemed that way. I do get angry at the way IBS sufferers are treated, but I also know that the vast majority of these hurtful quotes are the result of ignorance rather than malice.

I am well aware that my own knowledge of, say, diabetes is dismal, and if I met a diabetes sufferer I might blurt out, "Can't you just eat half a Mars bar?" and wonder why I received a frosty response.

We need understanding on both sides. Non-IBS people need to try to understand that IBS is a complex, difficult, embarrassing and long-term condition that can be very painful. And IBS sufferers need to understand that if you don't have bowel problems yourself, you probably don't spend as much time reading and thinking about them as we do.

If you are a non-sufferer and you're reading this book because your loved one or friend has IBS, then I would like to say, "Thank you." You are showing that you care enough to try to really understand the problem, and that can be the difference between a helpful friend and a hurtful one.

Second disclaimer

Please don't hit people with bricks.

No, it's all in *your* head

Some myths die hard, and some need killing. So before we move on, let's kill off the "all in your head" myth right here, right now. Let's destroy the fantastically moronic idea that IBS is all in the mind, that you are imagining it, or bringing it on yourself by being uptight and highly strung, and that if you just tried not to think about it then it would go away, magically, like fairy dust blown softly from the palm of a goblin's glove.

There are many reasons why this particular myth needs killing. First and foremost, it just isn't true. Scientific evidence now proves that IBS is not a psychological problem.

It isn't even true to say that IBS is caused by stress. Of course IBS is affected by stress, just like many health problems. The difference is that if someone has an asthma attack triggered by stress, his friends and relations don't immediately decide that stress is the sole cause for the asthma—but for some reason they do decide that for IBS. There's no research to support this idea, and plenty of research to refute it.

Another aspect of the "all in your head" theory, the idea that IBS is caused by neurotic obsession over bowel habits, is even more ridiculous. Now, I think about IBS a lot, even when I'm not writing a book about it. Some of the thoughts are practical ones about food or whether I'm well enough to go out that day, but sometimes I just think about it in general, like most sufferers do. If I had a broken foot I'd probably consider it from time to time; if I had a hole in my head I might give it a passing thought.

But here's a funny thing: Before I started suffering from bowel problems, I never thought about my bowels at all. No one causes IBS by being bowel-obsessed. The so-called obsession is the result of our condition, not the cause. And no one causes IBS by being anxious and worried, either. Yes, we *are* often anxious and worried. So would you be if there was a good chance of crapping your pants in public, or if your health for the entire day depended on whether you had been to the bathroom in the morning. But the IBS makes us anxious, not the other way round.

Stress and neurosis are the cover-all terms for any condition that the doctors can't explain. You blame the sufferer for his own condition, and there's your easy answer. It's not the doctor's fault for failing to have any insight; it's the patient's fault for being deranged. Doctors blamed stomach ulcers on stress for years until somebody pointed out that they were actually caused by a bacterium.

Saying that it's all in the mind is a semipolite way to tell the IBS sufferer that he needs to pull his socks up, grit his teeth and get on with life like a man. It's ridiculous for two reasons. First, it's from the school of thought that says mental health problems are caused by a lack of willpower and an innate character weakness (everyone with depression, for example, should take a brisk jog and get over themselves). Second, IBS isn't even a mental health problem to begin with.

Finally, what ticks me off the most is that anyone who insists that my symptoms are all in my mind is unilaterally diagnosing me with a mental illness, despite not knowing anything about my actual mental health.

There is—or should be—no shame at all in having a mental illness. However, I strongly object to being diagnosed with a mental illness when I don't have any *symptoms* of a mental illness.

I'm not depressed. I don't hear voices, I don't behave outside of social norms (most of the time), and I don't have breakdowns. I know my name and the year that I was born. I'm no doubt as eccentric and quietly odd as the next person, but I don't have any signs of mental illness. Except, of course, my malfunctioning gut, which is a sign of mental illness in itself. Right?

This is completely, utterly ludicrous. You might as well diagnose me with IBS if I've been having hallucinations but no gut symptoms; it's about as reasonable as diagnosing me with a psychological problem when I have gut pain and no psychological symptoms. Or diagnosing me with lung cancer because my foot hurts, or gout because my cat hurts.

We end up with a situation where our doctors decide that we IBS sufferers have failed to spot any hint of our own mental illness, but they as doctors have reached deep into our psyches and have spectacularly diagnosed the problem that we didn't even know was there, hasn't shown up as any kind of mental health problem, and only produces symptoms in our guts.

Medical professionals then decide to treat the IBS patient's alleged emotional and mental health problems in order to cure the IBS. Even when patients protest that the emotions they are feeling are surely normal for someone in pain and that they had been perfectly happy before their stomachs started making them miserable, the doctor still wants to cure the perceived anxiety or depression rather than the intestines. And if the patient dares to protest or get upset, it simply adds to the evidence for psychological disturbance.

I call this phenomenon the IBS Catch-22, and it goes a little something like this:

Patient: Doctor, I have been in pain for so long with my IBS, I feel so angry/anxious/stressed.

Doctor: Yes, your anger/anxiety/stress is causing your IBS symptoms; perhaps you could consider psychotherapy/counseling/a fortnight in Barbados.

Patient: But doctor, before I began suffering from IBS I wasn't angry or stressed at all. I lived a perfectly normal, happy life. It's the IBS pain that is making me angry and stressed. Can't we look for a solution to the pain, not the resulting emotions?

Doctor: No, because it is your emotions that are causing your IBS.

Patient: But I've only become angry after years and years of suffering, after years of being told that I have to learn to live with it, after visiting twenty doctors and having nineteen of them prescribe Imodium. And there's no correlation between the strength of my emotions and the severity of my symptoms. My IBS is as severe today as it was ten years ago. It doesn't make sense.

Doctor: Ah—I see that you are becoming more emotional as we talk about this. Indeed, you seem very reluctant to accept the fact that your emotions are causing your IBS. This shows that you are repressing your feelings and is a further indication that your pent-up emotions are in fact causing your IBS.

Patient: So you are saying that my overly emotional state is causing my IBS?

Doctor: Yes.

Patient: And the more I deny this, and the angrier I get, the more it proves your theory?

Doctor: Yes, that's right.

Patient: But how can I disprove your theory if arguing with the theory proves the theory?

Doctor: You can't, I'm afraid. Sorry.

The IBS Catch-22 needs to be put out of its misery. The leading gastrointestinal institutions of the world, including the International Foundation for Functional Gastrointestinal Disorders, now state categorically that IBS is not a psychological or psychiatric disorder, nor a disorder caused by stress.

IBS sufferers must be allowed to express strong emotions, emotions that are often related to years of dismissive and inadequate medical care, without having their feelings promptly identified as a cause of their IBS rather than a result.

Just to deal the final blow to the "all in your head" theory, here are some quotes from the finest, most respected gastrointestinal institutions and experts in the world:

> "IBS is not caused by stress. It is not a psychological or psychiatric disorder. It is not 'all in the mind.' Because of the connection between the brain and the gut, symptoms in some individuals can be exacerbated or triggered by stress."
>
> —International Foundation for Functional Gastrointestinal Disorders

"The irritable bowel syndrome is not 'all in the mind,' even though test results may be normal."

—Digestive Disorders Foundation, U.K.

"Does stress cause IBS? Emotional stress will not cause a person to develop IBS. But if you already have IBS, stress can trigger symptoms. In fact, the bowel can overreact to all sorts of things, including food, exercise and hormones."

—National Digestive Diseases Information Clearinghouse

"It is important to note that IBS is not a psychological disorder."

—Canadian Society of Intestinal Research

"To date there is no single identifiable cause for functional gastrointestinal disorders. This ambiguity can cause significant frustration for both patients and clinicians treating these disorders. It can also lead patients to think that their symptoms are 'all in their head.' This is certainly not the case. The symptoms of functional gastrointestinal disorders are real and can cause significant impairment and quality of life issues."

—Northwestern Center for Functional Gastrointestinal and Motility Disorders

"Stress does not cause IBS."

—American Gastroenterological Association

"IBS is indisputably a physical problem. Simply put, the brain-gut interaction of people with IBS influences their bowel pain perception and motility. In a nutshell, the processing of pain information within the central nervous system varies between normal individuals and those of us with IBS, with the result that we can experience even normal gastrointestinal contractions as painful.

The interactions between our brains, central nervous systems, and GI tracts are just not functioning properly. We have colons that react to stimuli that do not affect normal colons, and our reactions are much more severe."

—Heather Van Vorous,
author of *The First Year—IBS*

"Functional gastrointestinal disorders are not psychiatric disorders."

—University of North Carolina Center for Functional Gastrointestinal and Motility Disorders

* * *

So the next time someone tells you that your problems are all in your mind, say, "What an interesting opinion! I didn't realize you were such a *brave* thinker—to disagree with the International Foundation for Functional Gastrointestinal Disorders *and* the Digestive Disorders Foundation *and* the American Gastroenterological Association . . ."

CHAPTER 9

New Job, New Home, Old Guts

LET'S GO BACK TO MY STORY, and the gluten-free diet and fiber/magnesium combination that seemed to be working so well for me. As long as I stuck rigidly to my treatment regimen, which had to my amazement been working for almost a year, I had very little pain, very little bloating and perfectly formed bowel movements. It was wonderful. It was unbelievable. My digestive system digested things! Oh, the unadulterated joy.

My job was also going rather well. I worked for a publisher that produced magazines for pre-school teachers, so I was often sent books or puppets or fluffy sheep from PR companies, and once we'd reviewed them in the magazine, I'd get to keep them.

My colleagues were all very nice people. I would buy them doughnuts and they were always very grateful. I would have to hide the fact that I never bought one for myself, but in all honesty giving up a few doughnuts in the name of gluten-freedom was a tiny little sacrifice for the wonderful feeling of good health.

Although I enjoyed my job, I decided that my main goal at this point was to get a new job which was (a) closer to my hometown in Hampshire, and therefore the support of my parents and friends, and (b) far less reliant on trips out of the office—I wanted to be able to sit quietly in a corner.

Although my intestines were standing up very well to everyday life, I really didn't want to do anything that might upset them. Traveling and getting up at weird times and eating different foods would all qualify as upsetting things. Why do this stuff if I could possibly avoid it? It was just asking for trouble.

So when I applied for a new proofreading and editing job much closer to my hometown, and got it, I was definitely pleased. I wasn't quite ecstatic, as I knew there was always a chance that the IBS would return at any moment, but I was still very happy.

I moved into a flat near my new job and started work. My new boss and workmates seemed very friendly, and the work was not going to involve any early morning starts or reporting from outside the office.

I started work a few weeks before Christmas. On my last day of work before the holiday my boss presented me and my colleagues with our own individual Christmas presents, and I thought to myself, *Wow, what a lovely place to work.*

About half an hour later my stomach decided to wake up from its year-long slumber, giving me some impressive spasms and pain. I persevered at work for the rest of the afternoon, said my goodnights and thank-yous for the presents and walked to the bus stop with my ridiculous stomach cramping and tensing and complaining.

One minute I had been thinking about how lucky I was to find this new job, it's Christmas and the birds are shiny and the sun is singing and isn't it all grand and la-la-la. The next minute I was wincing in pain.

I struggled a fair bit with my symptoms in the first few months of the job. Constipation, my old standby, would kick in, with all of its accompanying pain and discomfort. This would be the day-to-day problem, and every now and then a really brutal IBS attack would come along with extreme pain and cramps. The IBS monster was back.

So why did the IBS come back, so dramatically and so suddenly? As with most things to do with my illness, I didn't really have a clue. There may be some people reading this who are wondering if the stress of a new job and a new home caused the symptoms, but I don't buy that. I have felt fine through times of enormous stress and been left in agony after gentle hoovering of the living room. My IBS seems to have as much correlation with stress as it does with the color of my pants.

It is possible that the change in tap water affected me. I had noticed when I was still at my old job that weekends spent at my parents' house would upset my stomach, which I always ascribed to the tap water. I was drinking a lot of water to go with the fiber supplements I was taking.

Because my new job and flat were fairly close to my parents' house, the water supply was probably very similar in terms of water hardness and the level of chemicals used to purify it, and so if my parents' water had affected me it seemed logical that the water at my new home and workplace would have the same result.

Before you dismiss this idea as ridiculous, let me say that I have experimented with different mineral waters and they definitely affect my bowel. And it's hardly surprising, as the amount of minerals such as calcium and magnesium in different water types can vary dramatically, and these minerals are known for their influence on the gut.

Some areas have hard water and some have soft, and the mineral that is responsible for making water hard is calcium carbonate, known for its constipating effect. From what I could gather I had moved from an area with very hard water to an area with equally hard water, so in theory the water should have made no difference to me at all, but you can never quite be certain what minerals are contained in your tap water unless you test it.

Having said all that, the water theory might be ridiculous. I'm always coming up with a new theory to try to explain my symptoms, and I'm sure that most of them are completely wrong. Actually most of them are demonstrably wrong; otherwise I'd be cured several hundred times over by now. But I had to cling to any idea that might bring about some improvements, and if bottled water instead of tap water might help, surely it was worth a try. I switched to bottled water and felt fantastic for a month and halfway decent from then on, with some bad days and some good.

My symptoms had returned with such a vengeance that I decided to ditch the fiber and magnesium combination, but I continued with the gluten-free diet as this really did seem to help. In my last job I hadn't told my colleagues that I was a gluten-free zone, and this had led to a few awkward situations where everyone else in the office was eating pizza, and I'd have to make some excuse or volunteer for pain.

Because of this I'd decided to tell my new colleagues about the gluten situation, although not the whole IBS situation. I just said that I was allergic to gluten and they accepted this very easily. The only problem arose when my boss asked me what symptoms I suffered from if I ate gluten by mistake.

You have to think quickly in this kind of situation, and it's usually best to lie—I told my boss that I got a bit of a stomachache and changed the subject. Do you really want to see how disgusted people are when you tell them about your *actual* symptoms? "I get constipated up to my eyeballs and then have to crap for ten hours."

There are sufferers braver than I am who are willing to talk very openly about their symptoms. And what happens? People say, "Oh my God, don't tell me *that*! That's too much information, dude!" People recoil in horror, as if you'd just revealed intimate and deviant details of your mother-in-law's love life rather than some basic facts about your bowels, which, let's face it, we all have and all use on a regular basis.

We IBS sufferers must be some of the only people in the world who can describe our terrible pain and be met with disgust. I suppose that lepers don't go down very well at dinner parties, but they probably get a bit of sympathy. Not that I'm saying it's easy to be a leper if there are any reading this. Sorry about the whole limbs-falling-off scenario.

To be fair, there are some people who are quite happy to hear about your bowels, but this causes its own set of problems. There is always the chance that someone is going to make a highly embarrassing comment or ask you a particularly scary question right when you can't run away.

My boss eventually found out that I had IBS and was sympathetic and nice about it. But one day, in the middle of our open-plan office, she told me about her friend who had IBS and had to wear incontinence pants and would sometimes run out of the cinema. "And we would always know *just* where she was going! Is yours as bad as that?"

Time moved on. I started to see an osteopath for my back pain, which I was still experiencing from time to time, and the treatment helped to keep the symptoms under control. I had a few really bad IBS episodes at work where I would be in serious pain for an hour or so and then it would gradually wear off. When these episodes happened I would just get my head down and hope that no one talked to me while I was battling through. (There's a bit in Helen Fielding's novel *Cause Celeb* where a really drunk woman at a dinner party thinks to herself: *If I could just stare quietly at a piece of bread then all would be well.* That was how I felt for much of my twenties.)

There were times when I genuinely thought I would have to give in and go home, but I just about held on until the pain passed and I could function again. Every time this happened it used up a little bit more of my reserves.

One afternoon I was in quite a bit of pain and ended up filing a load of paperwork away in a completely stupid place because I was so distracted. My boss needed one of the bits of paper later on and I blushed through a shameful hour of searching through all of our files to find the thing she wanted. I made some excuse about feeling unwell, but my boss was still rather bemused.

But I would always try to struggle through, partly because I hated drawing attention to myself by going home sick in the middle of the day, but also because there are only so many sick days you can take before your boss gets annoyed and your job is in jeopardy.

I mean, how many sick days did you take last year? Actually, thinking about it, that's not a fair question. I presume that you have at least a passing acquaintance with IBS, so your answer might be a little skewed.

Let's ask a healthy person instead. Look, here's one now. How handy.

"Hello, Arthur. Thank you for walking past just when we needed you."

"My pleasure. Bit chilly out."

"Can I ask you, Arthur, how many sick days you took last year?"

"Well, I had two days off for a bad case of flu."

"Is that it?"

"Yes."

"And would you normally go to work if you felt sick?"

(Arthur looks puzzled.) "No, I would take a sick day if I felt sick. I believe that is where the name 'sick day' derives from."

"Thank you, Arthur."

"No, thank *you*."

There goes Arthur, with a grand total of two days off sick last year. Now let's ask an IBS sufferer how many sick days they usually take. Let's ask me, because I'm here already. Well, I usually take no sick days whatsoever. None. Diddly squat with invisible sugar on top.

Wow, I hear you cry. *That's even less than Arthur! How do you manage that?*

Because I go to work when I'm sick. I go to work when I'm constipated or bloated or in pain. My sick days can't be used because if I use one up today then what happens for tomorrow, when it's worse, when I can hardly breathe from the suffering and I've used up all my sick days?

I go to work every day. My sick days are today and tomorrow and the day after that.

In the two years I was in my second job I took two whole days off sick, and one of those wasn't even for IBS. I was very fortunate (I am about to be sarcastic) in that I had three or four really bad diarrhea and pain attacks on the weekends rather than on workdays, which meant I could lock myself in the bathroom without anyone asking where I was. You see my good fortune.

Anyway, things were okay, but not fantastic. I was keeping on top of my work and eating food and seeing my friends occasionally, but I would sometimes find myself sinking into an IBS pit of despair when the symptoms returned. There was always a lurking cloud just waiting to rain on me.

And there were occasional reminders that my dysfunctional intestines made me very different from other people. One day I was on a training course with a group of colleagues. The course leader told us that to reach the toilets you had to walk halfway around the building and through a security door. To get through the security door, you needed a photo pass. If we needed the toilet we were to go to the front of the class and ask for the pass. Only one pass was available.

All adults can control their bowels. And if you can't? Well, you go up to the front of the class, say to the course trainer, "I would like the pass for the toilets please, and I may need it for half an hour or so to allow this pesky explosive diarrhea attack to pass," walk halfway round the building, and get relief. Or you just keep quiet.

On another day at work I received an e-mail saying that the water supply was going to be turned off for two hours and the toilets would be unavailable during this time. The e-mail was sent at 10:30 in the morning and the water was turned off at 11.

These incidents would just reinforce my feeling that IBS was so invisible it was never considered. Lovely, fluffy people who would go out of their way to make sure that there was wheelchair access to a training room didn't think twice about telling a roomful of adults that there was limited access to the loos.

Even when I was honest about my needs, the response could be rather underwhelming. At one work event I was told that a gluten-free lunch would be provided; this turned out to be a plate and a pair of plain rice cakes.

I was just exhausted by the whole sorry business. By this stage I was 26 and I had been dealing with IBS for over fourteen years. Wasn't it time I found a cure?

I stayed in my second job for two years in total, weathering the symptoms with differing degrees of success, but eventually I decided to quit my job and try to manage on my own in self-employment. This was partly because the workload in the job was getting ridiculous, but it was also because the prospect of working from home was so attractive.

Although leaving my job would be a risk, I was already earning a small extra income from designing websites. I sat down and calculated the amount of money I needed to live on and whether it might be feasible to work entirely on my own.

I lived in a small, inexpensive flat. I didn't drive a car. I had no children or pets, I didn't smoke or drink, and I didn't go out very much. I was very cheap to run. The more I thought about it, the more I was convinced that I could pay my way through self-employment. If I could do all of my work over the Internet I would never have to worry about meetings or outings again.

I would be able to take days off whenever I wanted to (within reason). I would have unfettered access to a private, Sophie-only toilet at all times. And I would be able to completely avoid all of those grim, soul-sapping, exhausting hours when I would be in pain at work and I'd have to pretend that I was fine.

I couldn't imagine how I would get through another forty years of sitting at my desk attempting to look normal while my guts tried to eat themselves.

I needed a boss who understood IBS, and that boss was going to be me.

CHAPTER 10

Money Worries and Intestines in the Media

I SET MYSELF UP IN SELF-EMPLOYMENT, and I remain self-employed to this day. I consider myself extremely lucky to be in this situation, as I honestly don't know whether I could have held down a full-time job for much longer.

I'm never going to get rich, but I honestly don't care about that. My number-one priority for my entire adult life has been to get some control over my condition. Other people want a fancy speedboat or a house in Spain. I just want working intestines.

It's worth mentioning the financial impact of IBS, as this is a feature of the condition that is often overlooked. It's something in my "things not to think about" pile, because if I sat down tonight and made a spreadsheet of every penny I have spent on fiber and supplements and gluten-free food and hypnotherapy, I'd no doubt have a heart attack at the total.

I am grateful that I live in England and the National Health Service has paid for most of my doctors' appointments and tests, but my dad had to fork out for the private gastro specialist to bypass a ridiculously long waiting list. I haven't asked my dad how much he paid for this privilege in case he wants his money back, but I imagine it must have been at least several hundred pounds.

The amount of money that we IBS sufferers spend on treatments is phenomenal. This is due partly to the inadequacies of mainstream treatments, partly to the long-term nature of IBS, and partly to the fact that our symptoms can get so miserable we will try any old miracle cure to get relief.

My IBS has also influenced my career for as far back as I can remember. There's no doubt that some of my peers are earning more money than I am and flying higher. Perhaps if I had had the intestinal fortitude I might have been up there with them. It's an area of my life where I have to be careful to give myself enough credit. Sure, I'm no company director and I don't live in a big old mansion. But I've been ill for most of my adult life, and bearing that in mind, I've done all right.

You know what makes me happy? Waking up in the morning with no pain, going through the day with no pain, and going to sleep with no pain. There are few useful things that an irritable bowel can teach you, but I have learned the real value of health. Many people don't appreciate that until it's too late and they have lost it for good.

I don't know if you remember Ally McBeal, the neurotic lawyer from the TV series a few years back. One of her favorite things to do was bang her head comically against a door and say through gritted teeth, "I have my health, I have my health," and of course it was funny because having your health really isn't any use at all, and she wanted love and marriage and money and success on *top* of the working intestines she already had. She was pretty daft.

IBS Tales

Although most people in my life now knew that I had IBS, I had yet to meet anyone who admitted being a fellow sufferer. Because of this, I was longing to hear from other IBS sufferers to find out how they dealt with their problems and whether they found their symptoms as overwhelming as I did. I had read many books on IBS by this stage, and the ones that I'd read the most avidly were those that had first-person accounts of IBS from real-life sufferers.

These books were useful, but they only included a limited number of personal stories or brief quotes, and I wanted more. I decided that I would set up my own website, IBS Tales, to satisfy my need to connect with other IBS sufferers and to provide a testament to the struggles of sufferers everywhere.

The IBS Tales site was established at www.ibstales.com and gradually built up a huge archive of sufferers' stories. Reading so many personal experiences certainly helped me feel less alone. The site also reminded me that although non-sufferers can sometimes be insensitive about IBS, there are plenty of caring, loving people out there who just want to take care of us. Here's an excerpt from one of my favorite ever IBS tales:

"Three years ago I met Nigel. He knew nothing of my condition and on our first date didn't comment that I only drank mineral water. During our second date we ended up at his house at a mealtime—I couldn't not eat! He made no comment when I asked him for boiled rice, broccoli and a glass of mineral water, and he even had some boiled rice in his soup!

"I eventually had to tell him of my illness. He rushed off to get pen and paper, and he wrote down everything I could eat. When I next visited him he showed me a cupboard in the kitchen—he'd filled it with all the food that I could eat."

I included a short version of my own IBS story on the site, and I was amazed at how many people e-mailed me to say that they identified with my problems. A firefighter in the air force wrote to me to say that he was sick of his colleagues treating IBS as if it was nothing and he was tired of trying to explain his symptoms to people who didn't understand. Maybe if an air force fireman found IBS tough, then I wasn't quite as pathetic as I had thought.

Teachers and nurses and librarians and soldiers and students wrote to me to say that they experienced exactly the same pain attacks and battles with their digestion and they knew just what it was like to visit unimpressed doctors.

After having lived for so long feeling like the only person in the world with IBS, it was a huge relief to know that I was part of a massive, indeed disturbingly large, patient group, and that everything I had ever thought or felt about my IBS had been thought and felt before by countless others. My despair and unhappiness had been normal human reactions to years of illness.

The stories sent to my site showed clearly that IBS is genuinely a terrible, painful condition and proved that although it affects patients in different degrees of severity and in different symptom manifestations, it can easily take over your life.

I started to do some research into the prevalence of the illness that had isolated me for so long. I was stunned at the numbers. I learned that IBS is so common it affects at least 10 percent of the population in places like America and the U.K., and some estimates put the number as high as 20 percent. That's at least 6 million sufferers in the U.K. and a staggering 30 million sufferers in the U.S.A.

I also learned more about the individual manifestations of IBS. Although my symptoms of constipation, diarrhea and pain were fairly typical for IBS, many people suffered from diarrhea with little constipation (known as IBS-D) or constipation with little diarrhea (known as IBS-C), and some sufferers alternated back and forth between diarrhea and constipation, never finding a happy medium (IBS-A). These symptoms were found in both men and women, and many children were affected too.

People with diarrhea-predominant IBS could go to the bathroom ten or twelve times in a day, and those with constipation could go a week or more without a bowel movement. I classified myself as an IBS-C sufferer because constipation was my biggest problem, but I had a lot of sympathy with the diarrhea sufferers as well. Life was no fun whatever end of the scale you were on.

The various symptoms of IBS were being relieved with a bewildering array of treatments. Patients were prescribed antispasmodics and antidepressants and antidiarrheals and fiber and laxatives and every kind of potion under the sun.

Less fortunate patients were told to go to psychiatrists and counselors, or that there was no treatment at all for IBS and they would simply have to learn to live with it.

There was no doubt that IBS was responsible for an enormous amount of suffering, and there seemed to be very few people who were taking this suffering seriously.

Let's all talk about poo

Now that my website had been established I began to receive e-mails from journalists who wanted to interview me about IBS. This seemed like a good way to get some much-needed publicity for IBS and a chance to practice being unashamed of my affliction.

I did a number of different interviews for a range of publications, mostly women's magazines. IBS Tales was once mentioned in *Cosmopolitan* magazine, in tiny, sideways writing on page 280, an achievement of which I am very proud.

I was happy to discover that I was comfortable talking about constipation and diarrhea and all the rest of it without embarrassment. I think I had been experiencing symptoms for so long that I simply couldn't be bothered to be embarrassed anymore. If the journalists wanted to laugh at me then surely all that meant was that they were cretins for being so childish. Say it long, say it loud: I am constipated and I am proud.

The result of this little publicity surge was a few very good articles, a few decent articles, and the occasional rather strange article. One journalist decided not to bother sticking to things that I had actually said as it was more exciting to make everything up. I was surprised to learn from her article that I had been terrified of having bowel cancer, but now that I had cured myself completely with a gluten-free diet all I needed was a man to complete my life. I hadn't said any of these things, but never mind.

Most of the interviews went well though, and it was nice to be able to talk openly about a subject that I very rarely talked about offline. The journalists were largely matter-of-fact and mature about things, although I did have one poor lady who was taken aback when I mentioned incontinence and nervously tried to establish whether I meant urinary incontinence or bowel incontinence without saying bowel, poo or anus. (She eventually went for "back bottom.")

I even did a live radio interview, on an obscure digital channel, maybe, but still live. I was also invited onto *GMTV,* but I thought that the chances of me getting through that one without coughing up a lung were quite low, so I declined. All in all though I was pleased to get some decent publicity for IBS and to see that it was possible for me to admit to all kinds of taboo toilet problems and still feel like a worthwhile human being.

Once I had completed these interviews I began to look out for any mention of IBS in the media. In some areas, bowels were quite a popular subject. Women's magazines in particular had definitely realized that IBS is very common and that many of their readers must suffer from it, and so they often mentioned it in their pages.

What I did notice though was that IBS was only rarely mentioned in newspapers and on the telly, and there was no one with a public profile who seemed willing to admit to having IBS. Celebrities were lining up to disclose all kinds of medical conditions, from Alzheimer's to breast cancer to erectile dysfunction, but nobody was standing up for bowels.

I did some digging and found out that the wife of Kelsey Grammer (*Frasier* from the telly) had IBS, as did Denise Lewis, the U.K. heptathlete who won a gold medal at the Sydney Olympics.

However, my favorite discovery was that Cybill Shepherd was a fellow IBS sufferer. Now, the star of *Moonlighting* and *Taxi Driver* only revealed her symptoms as part of a marketing drive for a new IBS drug called Zelnorm and came out of the IBS closet in a fluffy press release talking about how much the drug had helped her. Still, she gave some quotes about her symptoms that were more honest than anything I had ever read from someone in the public eye, and this was coming from a lady who had kissed Bruce Willis and won three Golden Globes.

She said, "For years I have been battling recurring constipation, abdominal pain and bloating. Go ahead and laugh. We laugh because we're embarrassed. In order for us to get relief, we have to talk about our symptoms and stop suffering in silence.

"I have tried nearly everything: changing my diet and watching what I ate. I exercised regularly. I even tried taking fiber supplements and over-the-counter laxatives, but nothing helped with all of my symptoms.

"My doctor used to tell me it was all emotional and psychological. So I got a new doctor. And a year and a half ago, I was diagnosed with irritable bowel syndrome with constipation. It was a huge relief to find out that my IBS with constipation was not all in my head and that it was a treatable medical condition. My doctor prescribed Zelnorm and it has provided me with relief for all my symptoms. In a lot of ways, I feel like my old self again."

You might argue that the world has gone celebrity mad, which I agree with, and that plenty of celebs are vacuous talentless nonentities, which I also agree with (although that probably doesn't apply to Olympic athletes and award-winning actresses) so perhaps I shouldn't be looking to these people for affirmation, but we all need to feel represented in the world. If I watch telly and never see a single item on IBS, it's similar to never seeing anyone with my skin color: it makes me feel invisible. If you constantly hear about diabetes sufferers and asthma sufferers and the dangers of obesity, but never hear a word about bowels, you begin to learn that your illness is far less important than these other worthy causes.

Some people believe that the fashion for celebrities opening up about every last aspect of their lives is distasteful and emotionally incontinent, and would rather go back to the stiff upper lip days when no one talked about such things and kept stuff private. That's fair enough to some extent—Britney needs some Marks and Spencer pants as a matter of urgency—but there's a big difference between offering up every sordid detail of your life for dissection and being open about subjects that we should have been discussing all along.

And yes, the issues that celebs choose to talk about may just be whatever cause or charity ribbon is most fashionable at the time—*Gay whales against racism* as one satirist put it—or the one that helps the star more than the people (or the whales) who are suffering. But sometimes there is no doubt that a celebrity has really gone the distance to help others who are dealing with an issue that is considered untouchable. Can you imagine Julia Roberts standing up and saying, "Diarrhea is my downfall and my hemorrhoids have driven me to drink"?

Talk to a handful of IBS sufferers and you will soon find someone who has waited months, years or even decades before seeing a doctor, because society has proclaimed that bowels are totally taboo. Who does this help, exactly? What cause does this serve?

Even when we pluck up the courage to visit the doctor we can be so tongue-tied that we don't properly describe our symptoms, leaving ample room for misunderstanding and misdiagnosis. If we could leave our shame in the waiting room it would be so much better for our health.

And things can change. Breast cancer is now regularly discussed on TV and radio, but thirty years ago it was stuck behind a wall of silence where breasts were not to be mentioned, cancerous or not.

If we can get a few more Cybill Shepherds to speak out for IBS, the celebrities of this world might start wearing ribbons for you and me, and leave the gay whales to fight for themselves.

CHAPTER 11

On the Blog

AS PART OF MY NEW WEBSITE ADVENTURE, I decided to set up a blog. This online diary would help me track the efficacy of any new treatments I tried and let me express my feelings about IBS.

The treatment tracking was important because I had been very, very bad at keeping records of the treatments I'd used. I would just try something for a couple of weeks and keep using it if it seemed to help and stop using it if it didn't. This was always doomed to failure because IBS naturally comes and goes, and I could easily have stopped using a treatment that was working for me just because I had a random diarrhea attack while taking it.

In the end I mostly vented my feelings on the blog instead of tracking treatments—and there were an awful lot of feelings to be vented. I already knew that my IBS was huge, but after writing the blog for a while it was even more obvious that my wayward bowels had a massive impact on almost everything I did.

IBS for Christmas (2 December 2004)

Ah, the good old Christmas season, when everyone gets flu and acts like they're dying when they've been ill for two days. We IBS sufferers have been ill for years, but do we moan, do we whinge, do we dribble? OK, yes we do, and that's exactly what I'm doing right now (not the dribbling), but I think we have the right. Anyone with a measly little cold gets sympathy galore, but we get laughed at. Is that fair, I ask you, is that in the spirit of Christmas?

I had a nasty few hours yesterday when I was thinking, *Shall I go home? No, I can make it. No, I'll go home. No, wait, I can make it.* I eventually made it, but this is no way to live life.

Wishing for the stomach of an ox (21 December 2004)

Stomach feels a bit dodgy this morning. Nothing major, but enough so as you'd notice.

The trouble with IBS is that you get this a lot—days where you're not sure how your stomach is doing, and you have to carry on until it either seems OK or announces that it will shortly be voiding its contents whether you are near a bathroom or not.

I've often wished for a stronger stomach. You know those people who say, "Yeah, I've got a cast iron stomach, I can eat anything"? I wish I was like that. Imagine being able to eat anything you wanted, at any time. Imagine being able to go on holiday to wherever you felt like, to go on a plane for 14 hours and arrive at the other end completely untraumatized by your bowel.

It must be such bliss. Except it isn't, because people with cast iron stomachs take their bowels completely for granted. They've never had it any other way. But if I was offered a cast iron bowel I would love it and stroke it and never let it out of my sight.

Not a good week (9 April 2005)

Well, that was quite painful. After around six whole weeks of a perfectly normal, standard-issue stomach, I've just had a week and a half of swathes of pain and gut disasters. Lord knows why. I seem to be finally coming out the other side now, but that was really not a whole lot of fun. And the trouble is that once I'm in an attack there's not much I can do about it.

Generally I choose between going to bed and trying to sleep through it (that's if I'm not at work or on the bus or something, in which case I try to avoid sleeping unless absolutely necessary) or just carrying on as normal and trying to distract myself with work or writing an e-mail. Of course, if it's a really, *really* bad attack then these choices are removed and I have to go and sit in the bathroom whether I like it or not.

Perhaps the worst thing is that when I have an extended spell of feeling OK, like I did for those six weeks, I start planning what I might like to do. And then my IBS says, "Nope, don't think so, matey," and puts a stop to it.

Oh well. At least I'm OK today. I should thank my lucky sheep. (Thank you, Arthur.)

Intestinal distress (20 April 2005)

Feeling a bit more cheery now. Oh, the wonderful cycle of pain that is IBS. Stomach is still being slightly bizarre, but at least it has stopped being painful. If IBS was only about stomach discomfort and weird gurgling noises (like I've got at the moment), then that would be no problem. It's the *pain* that really grinds me down.

Luckily I don't get pain more than perhaps three or four days a month now, but my stomach does have a comprehensive range of oddities which it uses to fill the in-between times. Take yesterday for example. No pain, but for about two hours in the afternoon it felt like I had a balloon being inflated and deflated and then inflated again in my lower intestine. As far as I am aware I don't keep any balloons in my lower intestine, so God knows what was causing that.

I've also been getting these kind of mini spasms where I can feel a small section of intestine wake up, perform a high-energy section from *Grease,* and then go back to sleep again. I have startlingly original bowels.

IBS depressed (7 June 2005)

IBS has been pretty bad lately. The past week has included: perhaps one hour of fairly intense pain, at least six or seven hours of fair to moderate levels of discomfort, intransigent constipation on at least a couple of days, plus the usual bizarre intestinal feelings such as spasms and weird stuff. And this is one week of my life, 15 years after first having IBS symptoms. Fifteen years later I still have to struggle and crawl and battle through my life instead of living it.

And the world somehow expects me to do just that. It always feels like whatever pain I am feeling or whatever is wrong with my body, the rest of the world blithely expects me to just carry on, just get on with it. That peculiar kind of British wartime mentality that says we don't care if you've got a bayonet embedded in your spine, you're to carry on living and not complain.

If someone said to me, "Dear God, look at what you've been through, you deserve a medal!" I would be pathetically grateful. But no one ever does. They just expect me to turn up or earn money or be happy and then are totally bemused when I am not.

I've had a stomachache for 15 years, I have to spend hours in the bathroom, there's almost nothing I can eat without feeling ill, I can't travel, and sometimes it feels like someone is stabbing me in the side with a lance.

Yes, but why are you crying?

No fun (4 July 2005)

Had some pretty insane pain on Friday and then through the weekend. Was so bad Friday that I was actually swearing out loud, which doesn't happen often. (I am a good girl.)

Then today has been bad again, colon not working properly and feeling like a large mongoose is trying to make its way through my digestive system in the most convoluted manner possible.

Spent about half an hour this afternoon trying to decide whether I should eat a banana, because sometimes eating helps and sometimes it doesn't. Eventually decided not to eat the banana. You see how high level my life is? You see the subtlety of the questions upon which I must pass judgment every day? You see just how incapable I would be of anything resembling a normal life?

At least the mongoose seems to have got where he was going. Perhaps he would like a banana.

Learn to live with it (12 July 2005)

Feeling better again now. Honestly, it's like being half a normal healthy person and half a completely decrepit person whose intestines refuse to conform.

I suppose the key to sanity is to enjoy the good parts and accept the bad parts—but not too much. I worry when I hear that IBS sufferers are told to "learn to live with it." Of course, in a way that's exactly what we have to do, but that shouldn't be the *first* thing we are told to do, it shouldn't be the doctor's first response.

We should receive advice about diet, medications, fiber, support groups, clinical studies, supplements and hypnotherapy. Then, maybe, if none of that works, we should be told to learn to live with it. But only then. Otherwise we're giving up before we've started.

Day in the life (18 July 2005)

Got up at around 10 a.m. on a Sunday. Feel OK, no immediate stomach problems. Have breakfast and take soluble fiber supplement as usual. No urge to go to bathroom. Usually have urge in morning, straight after breakfast. If no urge in morning then will be no urge for the rest of the day.

Still no bathroom urges. Go to bathroom anyway as sometimes no urge does not mean no need to go to bathroom. Nothing happens in bathroom. Feel OK until about 12 p.m. Start feeling tightness in stomach and bloated. By about 4 p.m. feel tight around stomach area and as if intestines are tense.

Get through rest of day feeling grim. Go to bed. Wake up, have breakfast, go to bathroom a minimal amount. Still feel tight and tense around stomach.

Repeat over 1,000 days of my life, and as far into the future as you can bear to look.

Two thoughts. First, if you would really rather that I didn't write about my bodily functions and think it's all a bit disgusting, well tough—this is my life, this is my greatest misery, and who the hell am I supposed to talk to?

And second, I don't know how long I can keep doing this, over, over and over. I'm so tired of it all. And so unhappy.

Planning your time (24 August 2005)

Bad day yesterday, but feel OK today. One of the most depressing aspects of IBS, and one of the most insidious dangers to your social life, is its unpredictability.

People say to me, "We're going out on Sunday, do you think you'll be feeling OK?"

And I say, "If you can just give me a minute to check with my fortune-telling IBS frog I will let you know shortly."

If I could predict the future it would make so many things so much easier. Just the guarantee of a decent stomach for a day would make life much more enjoyable.

Cheerleading hedgehogs (13 October 2005)

I sometimes feel, with a condition such as IBS, that it is necessary to set up some kind of motivational system in your head to keep you going. I tend to think of this in terms of cheerleading, having a little voice in your mind that keeps saying, "You can do it, just carry on a bit longer" and "One more day and your stomach'll be back to normal, you'll see. Just keep going."

This constant need to drag yourself out of despair can get pretty draining. I imagine my little cheerleaders (who I have decided to think of as hedgehogs, rather than proper cheerleaders, as 16-year-old girls would just laugh at me, and hedgehogs are more polite) are exhausted by now.

"Just keep going," they are panting, "just a little while longer," and then they collapse to the ground, several of them get run over by a passing lorry, and I have to carry on with depleted hedgehogs and a more feeble voice of encouragement.

I'm not sure what will happen if I ever run out of hedgehogs. Hope is the last thing to die, they say, so maybe my hedgehogs will last for as long as I do. I guess I'll find out in the end.

Still collecting symptoms (27 October 2005)

Even after all these years my IBS can still surprise me. It's not sitting still, no way, it's evolving, it's creative, it's hip and trendy and right in the now.

I just had a particularly weird hour-long episode. It was about 30 seconds of fairly intense pain, then a dramatic and very audible gurgling of the gut, then a break for about three minutes, then another 30 seconds of pain, then gurgling, and so on, until after about an hour it managed to resolve itself into some painless diarrhea and that was that.

So what on earth was that about? My IBS episodes, the really bad ones, are generally about an hour of fairly constant pain, and they certainly don't come with three-minute gaps in the middle. What was happening in those three minutes? Were the little IBS bugs giving it all they had in the 30-second parts and then stopping for some tea and chocolate biscuits?

Completely bizarre. And depressing, because just when you think you know what you're dealing with, you find out you don't.

Where were you when Kennedy was shot? (9 November 2005)

Someone sent me an e-mail the other day which said something like, "I remember my normal poops like other people remember where they were when Kennedy was shot."

That line sums up a lot about the IBS life. Non-IBS sufferers probably wonder what this poop obsession is all about, but we IBS people know. Your poop very quickly transcends its functional, practical, waste-removing purpose and becomes an iconic symbol of everything that is wrong with your body.

When you look at your poop you are no longer looking at the corporeal results of your daily munching, but a fortune-telling oracle for your day. Liquid poop? You'll be back in the bathroom within a minute. Pellet poop? Those spasms are gonna hurt later. No poop at all? Well, it was worth a go, thanks for trying. Keep waiting, Sunshine.

And a perfect poop? You are a pooping master, you are an intestinal professional, your body is no longer a source of suffering, it is a finely tuned digestional machine. And everything's going to be fine.

CHAPTER 12

The Emotional Effects of IBS

MY FRUSTRATED, TIRED AND SOMETIMES BLEAK blog entries revealed that living with IBS for so long had affected my outlook on life. I was never the life and soul of the party, being a quiet, shy sort of person, but I wasn't usually cynical or dark, and yet some of the blog entries I had written while in pain were pretty angry and upsetting.

When I was going through a bad IBS episode I would get frustrated with small talk and niceties. I didn't understand how people could walk around with permanent smiles on their faces and laugh over the slightest things, and I started to resent people who seemed to have a much easier life than me. The irony is that IBS, categorically not a psychological disorder, is enough in itself to mess with your mind.

Sylvia Plath wrote in *The Bell Jar,* "I wanted to tell her that if only something were wrong with my body, it would be fine. I would rather have anything wrong with my body than something wrong with my head."

Now, if you had tried living in Sylvia Plath's head, you might have seen where she was coming from.

The trouble is, of course, that if the thing that is wrong with your body is big enough and ugly enough then eventually it will *give* you something wrong with your head. Not something so horrifying that you put your head in the oven while your children are asleep, not something that robs you of your sanity or your sense of reality, but a definite disconnect from those healthy whatnots who have never experienced real illness; a gradual accumulation of resentment and a draining away of joy.

I *envied* people all the time. I envied their ability to eat whatever they wanted, to get up whenever they wanted, to fly off to Spain at a moment's notice and still poop in an orderly fashion. A colleague once said to me that he had a cast iron stomach, and I said, "God, you *lucky* thing!" He probably thought I was crazy.

After all, most people don't spend years worrying about their stomachs, do they? And I'm prepared to place bets that the first thing my friends think about when they make social arrangements is not, *I hope I have a bowel movement beforehand.*

When I was in pain or my stomach felt tight and horrible, I couldn't bear to have people around me, so I turned into a loner to avoid having to deal with people when I felt terrible. I didn't go to stay with friends because I knew that I would get ill, and even though I'd told them about the IBS I'm sure they thought that I was odd because I never went to see them.

How on earth can you tell someone, "I'm sorry, I can't come to stay because I would get unbelievably constipated, or alternatively I would have explosive diarrhea and may well poop on your floor." It's just not the type of thing that people say.

I felt like people didn't understand what a strain it was to always be wondering whether I'd feel okay today or tomorrow, whether I'd get through that meeting or whether I'd spend the whole day feeling like my stomach was going to pop. It was such a drain on my resources to have to fight all the time.

There's a famous quote about Ginger Rogers that says she did everything Fred Astaire did, only backwards and in high heels. Well I did everything that other people did, I got through school and university, I held down a full-time job and cleaned my flat (sometimes) and cooked my dinner, but I did it while being ill, and having terrible stomachaches, and not knowing whether I'd have a bout of IBS so bad I wouldn't be able to walk two feet from the bathroom.

I've done exams in pain, job interviews, driving lessons, birthdays. I read *Moby Dick* when my bowels were killing me, I wrote an essay on the great American novel when my intestines were spasming around like dancing centipedes, I took a psychology exam when my stomach was making such a loud and inappropriate noise that the girl sitting in front of me kept turning around to see why someone was disemboweling a platypus while she was trying to write about Chomsky.

The thing is, though, that I really didn't know how to interpret these things, to judge how well I'd coped with IBS, all things considered. Did all of this make me a strong, brave, resilient-type person, or did it make me pathetic and weak for giving in so many times and moaning about it so much? Would other people have cried as much as I had and struggled as much as me? I really had no idea.

I often wondered how sorry for myself I was allowed to feel and how much credit I should get for battling IBS. On a scale of common cold to tetraplegic, where did my problems lie? And if Denise Lewis could win an Olympic gold medal as an IBS sufferer, what the hell was I crying about anyway?

There's no doubt that IBS had caused me a lot of pain and limited my life in many ways. But other people struggle with health problems and a whole range of other problems, involving everything from money and relationships to addictions and crime. They have drug-addled fathers and monosyllabic mothers, grow up in trailer parks and have to fight to be allowed to go to college. Millions of people live in abject, crippling poverty and people still starve to death all over the world. So what in the hell was my problem?

I couldn't figure out how much complaining I was allowed to do without sounding like a spoilt little brat who needs a slapping. It was so easy to compare myself to people who were healthier than me, who pranced about with their working intestines and functioning bottoms, and forget all of the people with health conditions that were twenty times worse than mine.

And it all seemed like such a waste of energy. What could I have achieved if I'd put all the energy I had used to fight IBS into my career, or my social life, or some big overarching mega-project? A better job, more friends, a decent hobby? A shed full of paintings or a small troupe of trained cheerleading hedgehogs?

Instead, I had nothing to show for it. Every time I survived an IBS bout I had just survived, and that was all. I didn't even get credit for that, as most people didn't seem to believe that IBS was difficult to live with. So I got through another episode, and looked forward to the next one, and the next one, and the next . . .

I could go on and on and on about this, but I have to go to the bathroom.

Alone in the bathroom

I also struggled with a sense of isolation from other people. Not only were they all flaunting their own perfect digestive systems, they were also forgetting that I was not like them.

Every time someone who knew that I couldn't eat gluten offered me a sandwich or a pizza, I would get upset. Not outwardly. I just said, "Well that's very nice of you, but it might kill me, so I'll say no."

But inside I was thinking, *God, it must be so nice to be able to forget about IBS.* Or, if I was very grumpy indeed, I was thinking, *Can't you be bothered to remember that I'm ill? I have to think about it all the time, I have to deal with the suffering every day, the least you could do is not feed me things that make me sick.*

It's easy to forget the details of other people's lives, though. After all, who am I kidding? If I had been given a pop quiz about every aspect of my friends' experiences, would I really do any better? Of course not. We are all the center of our own lives, and we all have a number of different people around us jostling for attention. I really shouldn't have been so sensitive, but all the years of pain had thinned my skin.

I'm not even sure what I wanted. Did I want people to ask how I was feeling every single time they saw me? Did I want to give constant updates about the state of my intestines? I think I simultaneously wanted much more attention and sympathy and to be left entirely on my own. I obviously wasn't easy to please.

I often chose to be alone, sometimes reluctantly, sometimes not. It was a Catch-22 situation. If I socialized then I had to be prepared to turn down pizza and sandwiches and McDonald's and explain my reasons. Or I had to listen to all the wonderful things that my friends had been up to and then, when the conversation turned to me, tell them about the time I put the trash out.

If I didn't socialize I would just sit at home, trying to distract myself from whatever symptoms I had at that moment. If I didn't talk to my friends for a while I felt guilty for being boring and distant, and then I worried about losing them completely.

Just deciding whether or not to go out was a mini trauma in itself. A friend would invite me to dinner and my immediate thought would be that I couldn't go because my bowels were terrible and my stomach hurt, but then I would think that maybe I should make the effort, maybe I should say, "Sod the IBS and let's just go."

If I took a laxative I might be able to make it, but then I might be in more pain tomorrow from the laxative effects. Maybe I could just grit my teeth for one night? Had I got the strength left for one more night after so many years of IBS? And if I don't go to dinner, what do I say? That my stomach is killing me? But my friends must think I'm lying. I've had 429 stomachaches in the last five years and that doesn't sound very credible. And if you try a new excuse, like your cat ate a pillow and needs round-the-clock care, they don't believe you.

Life was full of these kinds of decisions, where I had to balance what my stomach wanted to do against what my heart wanted to do. My stomach usually won. I didn't often go out to dinner.

Where would I be without it

I would get upset when I heard about how well my peers from school and university were doing in their lives. Of course, I wished for them only good things, but sometimes I couldn't help but think that they had an unfair advantage.

These days you can read all about the lives of your old friends on websites like Facebook, and I'm often struck by the things that people choose to say and not say. Almost without exception the entries talk about jobs, spouses, children and all-round success in life, and not *once* do they mention dodgy bowels. I mean, *honestly.* Looking through these sites you get the impression that everyone else is ridiculously successful and accomplished, and there you are stuck on the toilet.

Of course, these little snippets of people's lives are highly edited versions, and if you could read the unvarnished truth it would include herpes and impotence and enormous throbbing piles, but the fact that you never do read about these things is another small reminder that IBS is nothing to be proud of, and the huge chunk of my life that has been dedicated to it is apparently worth nothing compared to careers and children and money.

There was no doubt that IBS had held me back. I'll never know for sure, but I like to think I would have gotten better marks in my school exams if I hadn't had to do some of them in pain. I like to think I would have been more successful in my jobs, been happier at university, been more stable in my friendships. I *know* that I would have been less of a grump.

Class of '96 Newsletter

Oliver and Samantha have bought a mansion in the suburbs and are expecting their third perfect child. Max proposed to his childhood sweetheart and is blissful on his honeymoon in paradise. Michael is President, Jemima is God, and Stefan won the Nobel Peace Prize. Sophie is trying to poo.

There were times when I felt like I had to turn off my brain because if I thought about my guts for one second longer I might marry a mauve hot-water bottle and move to a mud hut in Penge. I might, in other words, go a bit strange.

Looking on the bright side

Every now and then I would decide that I needed to cultivate a much more positive attitude to the whole bowel business. We are, after all, constantly told by self-help gurus that it doesn't matter what happens to you, it is how you deal with it that counts. In other words, if you have a great big pile of lemons then you better start making lemonade.

In some ways I see the logic of this. Most of us don't feel better if we sit at home and mope about our misfortunes. When I was miserable about my IBS I usually slept a lot or sat around watching telly and eating chocolate. This did not cheer me up. Surely I would be better off paragliding?

I do think that it's important to keep a sense of perspective about IBS. Someone once said to me, "Well, there are worse things than IBS," and although I wasn't terribly impressed with this comment at the time, it is true.

No one dies from IBS. It doesn't cause physical damage. It's not progressive. I can walk and talk and feed myself. There are plenty of people who are much worse off than me.

On the other hand, this positive attitude stuff can go too far. Sometimes "having a positive attitude" is code for "being in complete denial," trying to think positively about a situation that deserves nothing but negative thoughts. IBS is painful and grim and difficult, and I wish I had never ever heard of it. Is it really possible to be positive about IBS?

Sample chirpy journal entry:

> *I had a splendid attack of explosive diarrhea this morning which I very much enjoyed; the feeling of randomly spasming intestines continues to be wildly erotic. In the afternoon I laughed and laughed as I attempted to pass an extraordinarily large bowel movement without shredding my favorite melon-sized hemorrhoid.*
>
> *The absolute highlight of the day occurred on the way home when I experienced some frightfully enjoyable fecal incontinence just outside of Slough. You would not have believed the smell—my husband was almost retching it was so pungent. Another magical day!*

CHAPTER 13

Food Intolerance and Bad Bugs

MY SYMPTOMS STAYED MUCH THE SAME AS EVER. I was still prone to constipation, and the slightest change in diet or routine would initiate a constipation cycle that lasted for a couple of days. Every now and then I would get a diarrhea attack. Both the constipation and the diarrhea would be accompanied by pain or discomfort, ranging from bloating and fullness in my abdomen to feeling like a knife was cutting my guts.

Life in general was much easier because in my new role as a fancy-free self-employed Sophie I didn't have to worry about what my colleagues thought when I spent too long in the bathroom or try to act like a normal person when I felt like crap. But there were still a lot of limits to my happiness.

I had now been a card-carrying IBS sufferer for more than fifteen years, and I knew I couldn't go on like this for the rest of my life. I decided to dedicate my time to researching possible treatments and trying to find something that would help me. Thankfully I had a lot more time on my hands now that the daily commute had gone and I could work whenever I chose, and I became determined to use that time to finally find a solution, or at least half a solution. I started to read up on all kinds of different treatments for IBS.

I vaguely considered going to a GP and asking for a referral to another gastroenterologist, but all of the doctors I had seen before had been so utterly pointless that I couldn't quite bring myself to do it. It wasn't as if they had access to specialist drugs for IBS and they didn't have a set course of treatment for it either, so it seemed to me that more often than not they saw IBS as basically untreatable.

I wanted to find someone who genuinely believed he could help me rather than labeling me an entirely hopeless case, someone who understood how difficult it is to cope with IBS, and how impossible it is to learn to live with it, someone who didn't make a career of saying, "Hello, just going to put my finger up your rectum. It's IBS. There's no cure. NEXT!"

IBS Audio Program 100

The first thing I decided to try was the IBS Audio Program 100, a CD hypnotherapy program developed by one of the U.K.'s leading IBS hypnotherapists, Michael Mahoney. This program is rather famous in the online IBS community and I had read a number of stories from fellow sufferers who said that it had helped them.

My previous brush with hypnotherapy had not been an unadulterated success and hadn't relieved any of my symptoms. I had a sneaking suspicion that I was either immune to the hypnotherapy itself or that my symptoms were more closely linked to my diet than anything else. Still, I wanted to at least give the IBS Audio Program a chance. One of the reasons why I was happy to do so was that Michael Mahoney was honest about the fact that hypnotherapy doesn't work for everyone, because some sufferers will have food intolerances or other issues that need attention. This was a guy who knew that IBS is a complicated beast.

The program was easy to use. You listen to one session of hypno every day for 100 days (with some days off) with each session lasting about twenty minutes. I listened to the sessions at bedtime, and they were very calming and relaxing. I thought once again that hypnotherapy would be a great help for someone whose symptoms were triggered by stress.

I decided not to write about the sessions on my blog as the advice from

Michael was not to overanalyze my progress. I did have a symptom chart to fill in at the start and the end of the therapy, but apart from that I just ticked off a session a day and got on with my life.

At the end of the 100 days I evaluated my progress, and unfortunately the hypnotherapy had had no discernible effect on my symptoms. Looking at my symptom chart, I rated my symptom levels as being exactly the same at the end of the program as at the start: mild to moderate diarrhea, severe constipation, severe problems with alternating bowel movements, moderate to severe cramping/pain, mild bloating and mild pain in the rectum (ah, it's a glamorous illness isn't it). No real change in symptoms meant that this wasn't the treatment for me.

Food intolerance and bacteria

Next on my list of things to investigate was an IBS therapist I had found who believed that IBS is caused, in most cases, by either food intolerance, a bacterial imbalance, parasites or a combination of all three. Now, I don't really know if I agree with this viewpoint. There's no doubt that diet can affect IBS, and there's been some research to show that small intestinal bacterial overgrowth (SIBO) could be a cause of at least some IBS cases, but most theories about the causes of IBS are controversial and need lots more research.

To be honest, though, it didn't really matter whether I agreed with the therapist's ideas or not. I mean, I wasn't about to give good money to someone who thought that IBS was caused by an assortment of crochet teapots lodged deep in my colon, but on the other hand, all I really cared about was getting better.

Now, I do think, overall, it is vital to find out what causes IBS and to discover scientifically why certain treatments work. On an individual basis however, if it makes me feel better I really don't care why it works, as long as it does, and that applies to all you guys, too. If your favorite therapist claims to fish out the crochet teapots from your guts and you are thereafter cured forevermore, that is fine by me.

You should, of course, still be careful when choosing an alternative or complementary therapist because there are some truly ridiculous claims out there, and some very unscrupulous people who see difficult-to-treat, long-term health conditions as a quick and easy way to lazy riches.

I sometimes receive e-mails from people who, out of the pure kindness of their hearts, want to cure me, and the methods they wish to use can be jaw-droppingly hilarious. My favorites so far include wearing a magnetic bracelet that would do something miraculous to my energy fields and undergoing counseling to rid myself of the "anger at the family" that is apparently the root cause of IBS. (These e-mails from quacks are almost as welcome as the people who occasionally let me know that they really appreciate my website in a, well, *adult* kind of way, and would I like to correspond with them on this matter? I swear that's true.)

A few quick tips to spot a quack:

- anyone who uses the word "cure"
- anyone who uses the same treatment for a long list of illnesses
- anyone who diagnoses the same illness for a long list of symptoms, and so every patient who walks through the door coincidentally suffers from candida, which the therapist just happens to specialize in
- anyone who believes that IBS is caused by pent-up emotions or emotional tension or any other nebulous and conveniently impossible to quantify psychological problem
- anyone who gets annoyed when you ask for the slightest wisp of verifiable proof

Anyway, the ideas of the therapist I had found seemed fairly sound, and as part of his treatment methods he used some respectable tests to try to find out what was actually going on in an IBS sufferer's guts. I think it was the tests that won me over. Knowledge is power after all, and if something, for once, showed up as an abnormal test result then that was going to make my day.

The first step was to have a consultation with the therapist. I'll call him Ben, because I feel like it. I took the train up to London to see him and he was kind and polite. He listened to all my symptoms and then said he thought that the food poisoning I had suffered from when I was 12 was key to my symptoms (I wholeheartedly agreed with that) and that I probably had some bad bugs in my system that were causing the problems (I wasn't so sure about that part, but it seemed perfectly possible).

He told me what tests he was planning to use, what treatments he could offer, and that he was confident he could help me. I remember saying, "Wow, no one ever says that!" because no one ever had. Doctors were usually careful to say there wasn't much they could do and it was up to me to get used to it. I actually came *out* of this consultation feeling better than when I went *in,* which, if you are an IBS sufferer who's visited a number of healthcare people, you will know is very rare and quite exciting.

This is one of the great strengths of alternative practitioners. They are often far more optimistic about the possibility of positive results than mainstream doctors. That, of course, makes the patient feel great rather than utterly hopeless, and that feeling is worth something in itself.

The downside to this is that some practitioners go completely over the top and start claiming they can cure everyone and everything, entirely losing track of reality. It's a difficult balance between giving a patient something to believe in and offering false hope.

Ben seemed genuinely convinced that he could help me, however, and as his theories seemed so reasonable and I was very interested in the test results I decided to go ahead with his treatment plan.

ELISA food-intolerance testing

The first step in Ben's plan involved taking a food-intolerance test known as the ELISA test. ELISA stands for enzyme-linked immunosorbent assay, just so you know, and it measures the level of so-called IgG antibodies found in a blood sample when the blood is exposed to various foods. The theory is that if a certain food leads to the production of very high levels of IgG antibodies, then it could be causing your symptoms and should be excluded from your diet.

Blood tests for nut and other allergies work on the same principle but they measure the level of IgE antibodies, not IgG. In general the IgE tests are completely accepted by mainstream medicine and the IgG tests are more controversial, with some doctors arguing that the tests can give false positives to foods we eat on a regular basis. The tests do have their supporters though, and I was keen to find out my results.

Taking the test was pretty simple. I was given a home test kit that contained all the equipment I would need to slice my finger open and funnel half a pint of blood into a beaker. Wait, that's not quite right. I actually used a little "lancet" to produce a pin-prick of blood on my finger and a tiny vial to collect the blood.

It took me a few minutes to get the blood to go neatly into the vial, and I had to prick my finger about five times in order to extract enough blood, but it was basically an easy procedure and after I'd regained consciousness I popped the vial into an envelope and sent it off to the lab.

The results came back very quickly. Foods were split into one of three categories, color-coded red, amber or green, to show which foods you should avoid (red), which were borderline (amber), and which could be eaten freely (green). The results also reported, for the "avoid" foods only, exactly what level of IgG antibodies were found. The higher the IgG level the more significant the reaction.

My "avoid" foods were (with the IgG level in brackets): soya bean (15), rye (18), barley (14), wheat (14), rice (13), cow's milk (99), egg white (35), goat's milk (29), egg yolk (13), cola nut (65), pear (18) and Brazil nut (13). I also had amber (borderline) results for corn, peppercorn, coffee, grapefruit, almonds and cashew nuts.

So what did all of this mean? Well, obviously the first thing it suggested was that I should stop drinking cow's milk immediately. My result of 99 for cow's milk was far higher than every other level, and Ben said that it was one of the highest results he had ever seen. If I was going to give up milk, that would mean giving up cheese, yogurt and all other dairy products. That wasn't going to be easy, but it would be worth the bother if it helped me get better.

Although these results were useful on their own I was glad that I had a helpful Ben standing by to give me guidance. I mean, what on earth is a cola nut when it's at home, or even when it's on holiday? And did I need to avoid all the borderline foods as well or could I eat some of them occasionally? (It was decided that, if possible, I should steer clear of the borderline foods altogether to be on the safe side.)

I was quite happy with these results, although the milk thing looked like it was gonna be a pain in the bum. I was a bit confused though. As far as I knew I had never had goat's milk in my life, so were those specific antibodies just hanging around on a whim, waiting for an opportunity to strike? And could my extreme reaction to cow's milk simply be explained by the fact that I drank it every day without exception?

The ELISA test, as I've mentioned, has its supporters and its detractors, and there are those who believe that it is based on junk science and those who believe it's a breakthrough. At this point in time all I really cared about was this neat list of foods that told me exactly what I should eat to get better.

Comprehensive digestive stool analysis, or kindly crap in this small cardboard tray

(Do not read this if you're eating. I mean it. You have been warned.)

The second test that Ben wanted me to take was a comprehensive digestive stool analysis (CDSA) test, which checks for little bugs and beasties like unfriendly bacteria and parasites and also gives a general indication as to how well you are digesting your food. It is a pretty unpleasant experience, to put it mildly.

You are given a home test kit, which you use to collect three samples of your excrement over three consecutive days. This involves carefully pooping into a small cardboard tray and using a little spoon to collect samples of the poop. The samples are placed in a plastic tube of preservative liquid, you stir the mixture with the spoon, and then you shake the tube to make sure that the poop has dissolved. (I did warn you about the eating thing. Did you think I was kidding? Oh no.)

You then write your name on the tube, put it in a plastic bag, repeat the poop-collecting exercise for the next two days and send the tubes in a padded envelope to the lab. (Wouldn't you kill to be the postman at that place?)

I was a little worried about the "poop from three consecutive days" aspect of this test, as the main reason I was taking the test was to find out why I was so incapable of pooping on three consecutive days, but luckily I managed it this time.

The whole thing was undeniably disgusting, but at least it was hopefully going to provide some interesting information about the contents of my gut. And if my life ever depended on my ability to poop in a tray, I knew I'd be fine.

This is what the CDSA results showed:

Parasites—none found. This was good news as parasites such as *Blastocystis hominis,* which can produce IBS-like symptoms, can be very difficult to eradicate. They can also be hard to detect, but I was hoping that the CDSA test was accurate enough to find any bugs that were there.

Yeast/candida—none found. This was also good news as an anti-candida diet is very strict and dull. To be honest I'm not even slightly convinced that candida has anything to do with IBS symptoms, partly because it seems to be one of those diagnoses that alternative practitioners hand out to everyone they ever come into contact with, and partly because there's been no research to prove that candida has any relation to IBS. But apparently I didn't have a problem with it anyway.

Friendly bacteria—I had fairly low levels of the good bacteria species lactobacillus and bifidobacterium. Not ridiculously low, but enough to show up as less than optimal.

Unfriendly bacteria—I had fairly high, but not ridiculously high, levels of the klebsiella and bacillus species of unfriendly bacteria.

General digestion—small amounts of meat and vegetable fibers were found in my stool, which indicated that I might have a deficiency of digestive enzymes or hydrochloric acid and pepsin. I also had low levels of n-butyrate, a short-chain fatty acid. A range of other digestive processes were tested, including the absorption of nutrients from my intestines, and these were all normal.

So there was nothing major found in the midsts of my poop, and certainly nothing to match the intensity of the ELISA result for cow's milk. However, there were still several things that Ben thought he could address in the treatment plan he was designing for me. (Just as an ironic twist, we were meant to discuss my treatment plan in person, but we had to do it by phone instead because I was ill from the IBS.)

The final treatment plan looked like this: I would take a digestive enzyme, a good-quality probiotic, a butyric acid supplement, a black walnut tincture and a berberine and grapefruit seed complex. All of these things together were designed to boost my digestion, kill off some of the bad bugs and encourage growth of the good bugs instead. I would also take a liquid form of magnesium to help with the constipation.

In addition to taking supplements I would tailor my diet to fit in with the ELISA results. This would mean going both gluten-free and dairy-free, which was a rather daunting prospect. On top of avoiding bread, pasta, biscuits, pizza and the rest of it, I would now have to cut out milk, cheese and yogurt, as well as anything that contained any dairy product in its ingredients. It sounded like a very restricted diet. Some of my gluten-free replacements for staples such as bread and pasta contained milk, so these would now be off limits too.

It was going to be a struggle. What's more, if I found that a dairy-free, gluten-free diet really helped my symptoms, I was going to be faced with a very limited diet for the rest of my life. But it still seemed worth a try. I was willing to give up a lot of things in order to reduce my symptoms and if that included cheese on toast, then so be it.

The foods that had come up with lesser but still significant reactions, like pear and cola nut, didn't worry me as I didn't eat them anyway for the most part. The only "avoid" food that I was worried about was rice because that was something that I ate every day, but again, if it got rid of some of the pain then it was surely worth the trade off.

I was daunted by the dietary challenges, but I was also excited to have a treatment plan that was based on some actual test results and analysis rather than guesswork. It felt like we were approaching the IBS scientifically for once rather than beating its head with a blunderbuss and hoping it fell down a hole.

I started on the new diet immediately. It proved to be a definite challenge, but I had help from Ben in the form of diet suggestions and recipes, and of course I already knew how to be gluten-free. Breakfast was the biggest problem as I couldn't eat any wheat- or rice-based cereal and I couldn't drink milk, so that ruled out every cereal-type breakfast you care to name. I started eating a banana each morning with a cup of herbal tea, which was boring but functional.

The other meals weren't so hard. I could still eat meat, fish, vegetables and fruit, and I drank water or herbal tea, with the odd soft drink for special occasions.

For a few months things went very, very well. I felt better in myself, as they say, and I had relief from the constipation. I didn't have any major cramping or pain sessions and things looked really hopeful.

After a few months on the new regimen, however, it was apparent that I hadn't found my longed-for solution. The constipation crept back in, as did the bloating and stomach discomfort, and I was soon back to my IBS self.

This was so disappointing. I had invested a lot of hope and energy in this new approach, and I'd really thought it had potential. In some ways I'd seen it as the last best plan to help me. There were, of course, other treatment options available, but this was the one I had invested my hope and money in. And it had failed.

The mainstream doctors had nothing close to a cure and now the world of alternative medicine was just as weak when faced with my violent IBS. My guts had defeated everything I had thrown at them for sixteen years. I had swallowed every laxative and supplement and diet and drug and then crapped them all out again in a bewildering variety of gut-wrenching ways. And I was in pain. Again.

CHAPTER 14

On the Blog, Part Two

MY LATEST BATTLE WITH IBS HAD ENDED in another defeat, so I turned back to my blog as a way to vent my frustrations and document the symptoms that were still blighting my life.

Why doctors make me angry, part 38 (27 March 2006)

I just received an e-mail from an IBS sufferer that said: "The last doctor I spoke to told me that it sounds like IBS and it's all in my head and I just need to change my eating habits and think I'm healthy and it will all go away."

Do you see the kind of tripe we have to put up with? Do you understand why we might get a little miffed from time to time?

My top-three worst kinds of IBS pain (19 April 2006)

THE AGONIZER: This is the absolute worst kind of IBS pain because it's the absolute worst kind of any pain I have ever had the privilege to feel.

The Agonizer tends to last for around an hour all told. It starts slowly, with a few stomach cramps and gurgles, but within about 10 minutes it will have transformed itself into cramping, stabbing stomach pains. After about 15 minutes of me rolling around in agony

I'll have to go to the bathroom and sit on the loo for perhaps another 20 minutes of agony. And then it'll wear off.

After I've been through an Agonizer session I'm usually thrilled to have survived it for about an hour and then depressed for about three days.

THE WAR OF ATTRITION: Although War of Attrition pain is not as bad as the Agonizer, it comes in a close second because it is just so relentless. It basically involves day after day after day of a cramp in my right-hand side that won't go away for love nor money. It often gets worse if I'm constipated or my stomach is generally burbling, and so if I haven't been to the loo for a few days, it can get pretty damn bad by itself.

But the real problem with War of Attrition pain is the fact that it goes on and on and on, steady as a rock, grinding me down and sapping my energy. Whatever I have to do in life, be it work or seeing friends or posting a letter, the Attrition pain comes with me, always there.

THE BALLOON EXPERIMENT: This form of pain feels like someone is trying to inflate a balloon inside my intestines just to see what would happen. It comes in at number three on the pain scale because it only tends to last for about 20 minutes and I get brief breaks for relief before the cramps set back in.

Balloon pain is quite mysterious because it never seems to be connected to diarrhea or constipation or any other bowel symptom. It just comes out of nowhere and goes right back into nowhere, like a thief in the night or a mole in my lower colon.

Arthur the oversensitive friend (6 May 2006)

I'm doing pretty well, although I had a slight blip on the radar last week. Nothing major, just a bit of a tight stomach and discomfort, and I've been fine again for the past few days. This little blip has reminded me of perhaps one of the most infuriating aspects of having IBS, and that is the extreme sensitivity of my digestion.

This means that my intestines don't want any kind of change, ever, and if I do change something then I should always expect a reaction. Here's a little metaphor to show you what I mean.

Imagine you have a friend called Arthur. Each morning you see Arthur walking along and you say, "Hello, Arthur," and Arthur replies, "Hello."

Then one morning you say, "Hi, Arthur," instead of "Hello, Arthur," and Arthur says "Hello" back, and you think that everything is fine.

But everything is not fine. Because Arthur has immediately begun to analyze why you said the shorter "Hi" instead of a full and frank "Hello." He starts to believe that this signifies the weakened state of your friendship and the fact that you really have no time for him anymore. Slowly the realization dawns on him that you thoroughly hate and despise him, you plan to stop talking to him shortly and you would quite like to murder his cat.

That's what it's like with IBS. You change one tiny thing in your diet and your gut goes, "Three gluten molecules and an atom's worth of cheese, are you KIDDING ME? Well fine, you wanna be like that you go ahead, but I want three and a half hours in the bathroom tomorrow and don't even THINK that I'm not gonna gurgle."

It's the pain that grinds you down (17 May 2006)

I've spent about four hours today dealing with varying levels of pain. Nothing mind-blowing, I'm not about to collapse in a heap, but it's still pain, and it still means that I can't focus on anything properly because I'm too busy trying to ignore my stomach.

It's worn off now, so I'm OK again, but it's reminded me of the one thing above all others that is difficult to cope with, and that's the pain. When you read about IBS in the media, journalists usually concentrate on how embarrassing it must be to have IBS, and sure, it's not exactly fun in that department, but if embarrassment was the absolute worst part of IBS, then I'd be fine.

The truth is that I don't really care if people laugh at me if I have to run to the bathroom, because I'm too busy worrying that I might not be able to deal with the pain. I don't really care if I have another excruciating conversation with someone who asks me what my symptoms are and then really wishes they hadn't, as long as I don't have to put up with another bout of IBS pain that's so bad it makes me want to garrote myself with the shower curtain.

And I could cope with the bloating and the weird gurgly noises and the rushing to the loo and the never rushing to the loo and the avoidance of all foods which taste like something I might ever want to eat if it meant that I would never have the pain. It's the pain that really saps my spirit; it's the pain that grinds me down.

Normal service resumed (4 June 2006)

Right. Finally I am again living in a world where men are men and intestines are intestines rather than instruments of torture. Hurray. I've been quite strict about keeping to a going to bed/ getting up schedule over the last week and that seems to have done the trick. It's still annoying to have to tailor my life around my stomach, but if it avoids the kind of experience I had last weekend then who really cares? It's worth it.

I got to the lovely stage where (this next bit is not to be read by people of a nervous disposition) it felt like the waste was actually crawling further and further up inside me, and my stomach was starting to feel like it would much rather explode than digest things. (Look, I'm sorry for being gross, but this is a blog about irritable *bowel* syndrome so I'm gonna have to talk about bowels. I wish it was a blog about ladybirds or something, but it isn't.)

This three-day constipation feeling is one of my most hated feelings in the world. It feels like my stomach is constantly tensed and there's nothing I can do to relax it. The only way I'm gonna get relief is if I go to the bathroom, and I have no way of knowing when that miraculous event will occur. Yuck, and, if I may say so, bleurghh.

Still, gotta count my blessings. I feel fine today, I felt fine yesterday and I might feel fine tomorrow. That'll do for now.

Invisible illnesses (11 June 2006)

Most of us IBS sufferers know the drill. You've been in pain for weeks on end, your stomach is killing you, and you go into the office or the classroom day after day after day and nobody offers to help you. And then some clown comes in with a cold and gets surrounded by well-wishers before he's even sat down.

And as if that wasn't enough he then milks it for all it's worth. "Oh, I'll struggle on," the guy sighs, "I'll somehow make it through." Because obviously he is so important that the whole place would fall apart without him, and he'll manfully find a way to cope with the incredible agony that comes with a blocked-up nose and some phlegm.

Humph, I say. And bah humbug. You know what the problem is? Invisible illnesses. If you get a cold, everybody knows about it because you sneeze at regular intervals. "Look at me, poor old me," say the sneezes. "Sympathy to come in this direction."

IBS sufferers just don't have a sneezy equivalent. Sure, sometimes you have to run to the bathroom, but people just laugh at that. Your greatest moments of agony are experienced alone, in a locked room, out of sight. Even when you're walking around in constant pain no one can see it, so no one offers to help.

If we human beings are the product of a higher power, then God must have been interrupted halfway through designing the pain signals. He had just decided that pain would be a great way to let us know that something needed fixing and then the doorbell rang, so He never got round to the second part: working out how to show us exactly where the pain was, and exactly how to go about fixing it.

If I have a stomachache then my stomach should glow bright purple. If my intestines are killing me, I want thick fluorescent stripes across my gut.

I'd walk into a room and people would turn away from the Pathetic Little Person with a Cold and gasp in dumbstruck awe at the Incredible Heart of Courage of the Fluorescent-Stomached Girl. That'd show them who deserved all the sympathy.

A wedding and a list of worries (18 June 2006)

One of my old school friends is getting married next month, which is obviously very good news and I'm very happy for her. Unfortunately, as a loyal and committed IBS sufferer, this wedding has given me a range of things to worry about because I can't just pop along to the church and then stroll casually over to the reception. Why?

Well, because I might be in pain. That might be pain that comes on for half an hour and then goes, in which case I'll be OK, and I'll grit my teeth and make small talk with random people and get through it. Or it might be mild pain throughout the day, in which case I'll grit my teeth and make small talk and then collapse in a heap once it's over.

Or it might be excruciating, mind-numbing pain, in which case I just won't be able to go. Or perhaps the worst kind of pain would be the pretty-bad-but-not-disabling kind of pain, where I'll have to make a decision about whether I should just not go or whether I should go in spite of it and pretend to be happy and healthy all day while feeling like I want to drop dead.

And then, of course, I might need a bathroom. I'm fairly lucky in this respect compared to other sufferers in that it's actually quite rare for me to need the loo after I've got through the first few hours of the morning, but it still happens sometimes. And any kind of public gathering of several hundred people is really not the place to get the runs. There'll be queues, and no paper, and people trying to pretend they're not listening as I flush 39 times and make highly inappropriate groaning noises.

And there'll be all those random people. I'm socially questionable at the best of times, but my bowels make it that much harder. I'm having a lovely chat about the flowers or the weather or my work or whatever and I watch in horror as the conversation steers itself to an IBS-related area.

"So why do you work from home?" someone will ask. Or "Hey, Bob said you run a website, what's that about?"

"Because my bowel likes to torture me with constipation that knows no bounds," I will reply. "And the website is all about poo."

Opinions to yourself, please (9 July 2006)

A fellow sufferer has sent me a great quote about some people's attitudes to IBS. She says, "When people say, 'Have you tried drinking more water?' or 'Maybe you just need to learn to relax,' in that patronizing and quite dismissive way, I feel like saying, 'Look, I don't say to you, "Have you tried wearing a more flattering shade of lipstick?" when you tell me you think your husband is having an affair.'"

That really sums up the attitude of some non-sufferers, for two reasons. Firstly, because for some inexplicable reason people often feel compelled to offer advice the moment they hear about your problem, despite the fact that their knowledge of IBS amounts to one tiny article in the *Daily Mail.*

And secondly, it shows the size of the gap between our own perception of IBS and the non-sufferer's perception. If your husband's having an affair, a bit of lipstick won't make the slightest difference. And if you have IBS, you have a serious, intractable, painful disorder, so why do people think it's so easily cured?

Tired (22 July 2006)

Intestines have been a bit dodgy for the last couple of days. I don't know why, but then I never know why, so nothing changes. For some reason I just feel exhausted today. Tired of having to put up with this stuff for 16 years, and tired of having to cope, but mostly just tired of wanting something so badly for year after year and never getting it.

There aren't many things I want in life. The other day I decided that the only things I really wanted were a flat of my own and one of those expensive reclining chairs that has a fridge in the armrest and does the hoovering while you sleep.

But I could live without those things very easily, and if I never get them then I won't really care. If I never get rid of the IBS, I don't know what I'll do. Fifty more years of this? I'm 28 years old and I'm so tired.

Pain in the arse (25 July 2006)

Over the weekend I developed a new and exciting symptom which I feel I should record for posterity. This new symptom has confirmed my belief that IBS is a vibrant, energetic, ever-changing masterpiece of a disorder. Not for me one of those stick-in-the-mud illnesses that gives you the same symptoms all the time, oh no. I have an illness that *evolves.*

And my new symptom? Bottom pain. Yes indeedy-o, just when you thought that cramps and spasms and constipation and diarrhea and bloating and agonizing stomach pain might be enough to be going on with, your body decides otherwise. And gives you a pain in the arse.

I can't tell you how thrilled I am about this development. What it means is that rather than just finding it difficult to go to the toilet on constipation grounds, I can now also appreciate what it might feel like if you tried to extract a wardrobe from your rectum. This is hugely useful knowledge.

Thankfully, after a few days of suffering I was able to visit the toilet this morning without the bottom pain manifesting itself. However, this presents me with another pressing problem, which runs thus: I'm actually quite happy this morning, but it's a fragile form of happiness. If I were to sit down and analyze the source of my joy it would soon disappear into nothingness.

No one wants their state of mind to depend on pain-free pooping.

Two weekends (14 August 2006)

The weekend of the guy who lives upstairs. On Saturday he wakes up with his girlfriend. They talk and giggle for a while (the ceiling is fairly thin, and the sound travels down). They make love (girlfriend is pretty loud, bed is pretty squeaky). They get up and clank pans around, laugh and talk some more, and go out at noon. They come home later, talk and laugh again, make love again and go out again at eight. They don't come home on Saturday night.

My weekend. I wake up on Saturday and feel fairly uncomfortable because I am constipated from the day before. I have breakfast and a cup of coffee, but when I try to go to the bathroom nothing much happens. This means that I have now been constipated for two mornings running, which means bloating and tightness and pain. I try to sleep some of the day away and don't do much in the evening. I find it difficult to sleep on Saturday night, and my gut feels congested and stretched.

On Sunday I wake up and have breakfast. I finally manage to pass a hard bowel movement by straining on the toilet. In the evening I am in the shower when I start getting some really vicious stomach cramps. After about half an hour of terrible cramps, I have another bowel movement. And then I feel fine.

Presidential piles (9 June 2007)

I stumbled upon a website the other day which lists the health problems of every American president (www.doctorzebra.com/Prez/t_roster.htm). Obviously the first thing I did was look for digestive woes, and, my God, did these men have digestive woes!

I've chosen some of the best gastrointestinal malfunctionings and listed them below. I have to say I find it quite cheering to know that you can be the leader of the free world and still have hemorrhoids.

Thomas Jefferson had life-threatening constipation after a severe illness.

Andrew Jackson had chronic abdominal pain and diarrhea for years, possibly dating from a bout of dysentery contracted from the swamps of Florida. Could this be the first ever recorded case of post-infectious IBS?!

James Garfield had an anal fissure which kept him in bed for several weeks and was operated on. He also had a "weak stomach" for years—was he another IBS candidate? And he was fed through the rectum following an assassination attempt in 1881. Don't really want to know why.

Franklin Roosevelt had severe iron deficiency anemia which was ascribed to bleeding hemorrhoids.

Dwight Eisenhower suffered from Crohn's disease and a bowel obstruction.

Jimmy Carter was forced to leave a Christmas party in 1978 "to receive emergency treatment for a painful hemorrhoid that left him almost completely incapacitated." He had first suffered from hemorrhoids as a young man.

Bill Clinton had a colonoscopy to investigate rectal bleeding, but nothing sinister was found.

George W. Bush had a hemorrhoid while serving in the National Guard and also had some colonic polyps removed.

And finally, **John F. Kennedy**. I've saved him for last because, as you'll probably know, JFK was almost frighteningly unhealthy. His list of malfunctioning bits and pieces includes a bad back which was so chronic he had to wear a back brace most of the time, and Addison's disease, an endocrine disorder that almost killed him.

For us intestinally demented folk, JFK's most interesting malady was a prolonged gastrointestinal problem, which was treated with steroids and at least three different antidiarrhea medications such as Lomotil.

The first record of JFK's digestive distress dates back to when he was just 17. Later on, when he was in the Navy, it's fascinating to see that his disorder was described as "severe spastic colitis"—the old-fashioned name for IBS. Was Kennedy one of us?

There's some speculation that JFK might actually have had undiagnosed celiac disease or an inflammatory bowel disorder such as Crohn's disease. What is certain is that he had some very nasty diarrhea attacks, and it is recorded that just before and just after the Bay of Pigs invasion Kennedy was suffering from "constant, acute diarrhea" and was treated with antispasmodics, puréed food and penicillin.

So the next time you're ill and some clown tells you to relax and stop worrying, say, "If the 35th President of the United States can't control his own bowel, then how can I?"

CHAPTER 15

Relief at Last

ALTHOUGH THE FAILURE OF THE CDSA and ELISA approach was a major disappointment, it had at least opened my eyes to some treatment avenues that I had not yet explored. The problem was that I hadn't come across any other approach that appealed to me. There were an awful lot of loopy people who wanted to cure me with crystals and healing energy and marshmallow enemas, and hardly anyone who wanted to use evidence-based treatments and science.

So instead of looking for another doctor or alternative health person, I started to analyze the times in the past when I had felt well, in the hope that I could remember the treatments I had been using and give them another go. The period of time that sprang to mind was what I had taken to calling my "mystery year," the time during my first job when I had felt very well indeed for almost an entire year.

I had started thinking of it as my mystery year because I could see no real reason why the symptoms had abated as much as they did. More importantly, I knew that I had used fiber, magnesium and a gluten-free diet and then abandoned the fiber/magnesium combination when the symptoms eventually returned regardless.

I had written off the fiber and magnesium supplements as just a temporary fix. But what if I had just been going through a larger-than-life IBS episode that would have resolved itself in time, and the supplements had been working nicely in the background? I began to think that I had stopped taking these products far too quickly, almost as if I was pessimistically convinced that nothing could touch my symptoms, when that was clearly untrue.

I decided to try the fiber and magnesium again. The trouble with this plan was that I couldn't remember exactly what dosages I had been using. I knew that I had been taking Normacol and Celevac for the fiber part, so I decided to start right away on the maximum daily dose of both. Technically us IBS folk are supposed to start taking fiber slowly and work up to the highest dose if needed, because a sudden increase in fiber can cause bloating and pain in some sufferers, but for whatever reason it's never had that effect on me.

The biggest problem was the magnesium. I knew that I had used magnesium citrate tablets, and I could even remember the brand I had taken, but I couldn't remember the dose. I thought it was probably around 450 mg a day, 150 mg in the morning and 300 mg at night, and so I started off with that.

I soon found that a 450 mg dose gave me diarrhea, so I tried 300 mg, and that gave me stools that felt like I was trying to lay a pineapple, and I couldn't try anything in between because I only had 150 mg pills.

I was stuck in magnesium trial-and-error land for quite a while. I persisted because of my mystery year memories, and also because it was so evident that magnesium had a tangible effect on my gut, which was worth holding on to: I had taken enough drugs and supplements over the years that might as well have been sugar pills to recognize the value of a pill that really got to me.

I kept experimenting with different doses of magnesium. I spent quite a few months taking 450 mg and putting up with being a little on the diarrhea side of life, because that was usually fine by me. As long as I was pooping regularly I didn't really care how quickly the poop exited or where it ranked on the Bristol stool chart. (Doctors use the Bristol stool chart to evaluate the relative perfection of patients' poops. There are seven levels of poopal variations, to cover anything from hard rabbit pellets to a fluffy soft mess. I don't know who invented this chart, but if we ever met in real life, we would have a lot to talk about.)

A little while later I decided to reduce the dose a little, and after much fiddling about, and a switch to taking both plain magnesium citrate tablets and magnesium/calcium citrate tablets, I settled on a regimen of 400 mg of magnesium citrate each day plus 200 mg calcium citrate. I also remembered that I had been taking vitamin D capsules the last time I used this regimen, so I added 400 IU of vitamin D in, too.

And miracle of miracles, I began to feel spectacularly, blindingly well. The mild diarrhea reduced, and eventually I even managed to produce a few of the splendidly formed bowel movements of yore. The major IBS attacks practically vanished altogether. I still had the occasional constipation situation but that was easy enough to deal with.

To my amazement, I began to think of myself not as an IBS sufferer, but as a fit and healthy person with a bit of a sensitive stomach. I began to take my successful digestion for granted, going on outings and booking appointments without worrying about the bowel side of everything.

I even found that my formerly rigid routine could be relaxed without consequences. I had stuck to more or less the same getting up time for years and years, and if I varied this by more than half an hour either way I was asking for trouble. But now I found that I could get up later and later without any problems whatsoever. One day I got up at noon just to test myself, had breakfast, and went to the bathroom like a pro. This was something special.

And this, amazingly, stupendously, is still the state of my bowels today. I have now had another entire mystery year of wellness, with much less mystery this time. In the past year I have had perhaps five or six days of constipation, a handful of days of other symptoms such as bloating or discomfort, and one or two painful cramping attacks. So that's maybe two weeks of symptoms out of twelve months of living, an incredible record for someone who used to go months without a break from her bowels.

I can't tell you what a relief it is to wake up and expect to be free of pain, to book appointments and meetings without considering my intestines first. What an incredible feeling it is to just sit quietly and not be able to *feel* my stomach. You probably need to be an established IBS sufferer to understand the joys of that one.

I am still amazed that this body, which protested so loudly for so long about the fact that I asked it to digest things, is now working so well. How can a digestive system that is capable of such dysfunction now function so smoothly?

I am incredibly grateful that I have been able to get to this point. There were so many times when I thought I was going to have to cope with IBS attacks for the rest of my life, and that was unbelievably daunting. This is *easy.* I often sit and think about how much easier my life is without the symptoms. Instead of having to crawl and batter my way through life, I can casually walk through it. I wake up with the assumption that I will be pain-free today and my body does not betray me. It feels like exhaling after years of holding my breath.

It has been months now since I have had to work around my IBS rather than making it work around me. I go where I like, when I like; I don't worry about the possibility of pain, because 99 percent of the time it doesn't exist. I can commit to events months in advance without worrying about whether I'm going to be well enough. I feel like a healthy person rather than someone who is consumed and defined by her illness.

I do still have limitations on my life, but I have accepted these. A gluten-free diet is not particularly easy to stick to, but it is much, much easier than coping with IBS. I miss French bread and doughnuts and pizza, but not enough to tempt me to eat them. In fact, I hardly ever think about my diet anymore because I've been following it for many years now and it's become a useful habit.

I am not cured by any means, but this is an IBS that I *can* live with. Maybe this is what most people and most doctors imagine IBS to be: a bit of diarrhea here and there, a bit of pain now and then, and nothing more. Anyone could live with that, but I found it almost impossible to live with IBS at its most vicious. If I am very, very lucky then I won't ever have to again.

The almost end

And that's my IBS tale. It's been a long, long story and it's certainly not over yet, but at least I'm still here to tell it, and I'm mostly winning the battle against the beast of my bowel.

After all these years and all these pages I have a little voice in my head saying that I should tell you how much I have learned from my, um, *journey,* and how much wisdom I have gained from all that pain. But I won't.

I know that many people believe in the power of suffering: they think it builds character, it makes you human, and it teaches you compassion and strength. But I think that's just one of those happy little philosophies we invent to get through the tough stuff. Can you imagine if pain had no point except to hurt you? Nobody could deal with that.

But that, generally, is what I believe. Suffering is painful and pain is pointless. Pain makes me miserable and useless and floppy, the limitations of IBS make me grumpy and caged and scared, and chronic illnesses wear us down to the point where we don't know how to cope any longer. You get rainbows with some of the raindrops, but mostly you just get wet.

You might well disagree with me on this, depending on whether you look for meaning in life's events or like to think that they're basically random. I prefer to believe that we are better off avoiding pain if we can possibly help it. It is quite painful, after all, and I can think of better things to do with my time.

One of the best coping strategies I have developed is to allow myself to feel aggrieved for a while, to go off in a great big grump and acknowledge that life has been tough for me sometimes, as it is for everyone, and that my feelings are perfectly normal.

A genuinely sympathetic friend will tell you that IBS sounds horrible rather than trying to convince you that it's nothing to get upset about, and we should do this for ourselves as well. We feel what we feel for a reason, and our feelings of despair are entirely valid. To believe anything else is to buy the old, old lie that says an irritable bowel is no big deal.

In fact, if I have one ambition for this book it is to tell the absolute truth about the power of IBS and to show how normal we *all* are when we find it so difficult to cope with. IBS is awful, and telling us to look on the bright side is just insulting.

However, I do need to acknowledge that there have been some positive aspects of my IBS experience. I care about my website, and I'm proud of it. I care about this book. These are ways that I have channeled my pain, I suppose, and made use of all that angst.

I'm very glad to have made contact with so many other IBS sufferers over the years, to have learned so much about their lives and their own coping strategies, and to hear how nurses and teachers and firemen and soldiers and technicians and writers and actors and school kids live with the symptoms I know so well.

My diet is lovely and healthy now that I can't eat pizza or chocolate cake and have to eat boring rubbish like fruit all the time. And I often think, *Wow, my stomach feels great today.* I can get a whole day's worth of good mood from that one thought alone. I doubt that many other people wake up and smile because they haven't got a stomachache. And that's pretty cool. Not worth twenty years of suffering, but cool nonetheless.

I may take some things for granted in my life, but not my health, ever, and that's not to be sneezed at. IBS may not have conferred on me any great wisdom or enhanced my spirituality, but it has made me look around and recognize luck and good fortune when I see it, and there's been a lot of it around me in my life.

I have accepted that IBS is a lifelong condition that will always be mine. I have had it for so long now that it's difficult to remember what my life was like without it. I have spent the whole of my adult life as an IBS sufferer, and the whole of my teenage life as well, and it is as much a part of me as my job or my color or my gender. There ain't nothing I can do about it, that's just the way it is. And finally, after all this time, that's all right with me.

My name is Sophie Lee and I have irritable bowel syndrome. What's your problem?

CHAPTER 16

Remedies I've Tried

I DON'T THINK MY STORY WOULD BE COMPLETE without a comprehensive list of all the remedies I have tried, just to show how many different treatments an IBS sufferer can go through before they find something that actually helps. There's a good reason why doctors don't get enthusiastic about their IBS patients: we're an absolute pain in the bum.

This list is also here to encourage you, if you suffer too, to take a good look at all of the remedies you have tried over the years, try to analyze what has worked, and then see what you could try for your next treatment. The point of this book is to tell the truth about IBS. The truth is that, to my amazement, I have largely put an end to my suffering, and I very much hope that you can too. My story is proof that the most delinquent of bowels can be tamed.

I do have to be careful here though, because it's all too easy for someone who's feeling well to tell someone who is suffering what to do. Indeed, there's a particularly annoying type of person, the medical equivalent of the Bridget Jones "Smug Married" type, who likes to lecture ill people about how quickly they could get better if they just followed the Smug Cured Person's advice.

I don't want to be one of those gits, so let me make it plain that I'm mainly writing this list as a record of my own treatment over the years. If something on it works for you, that's great, but I'm under no illusion that I've stumbled upon the Universal Path to IBS Wellness. I did come to my own good health through a torturously circuitous route though, and maybe I can offer you some shortcuts.

Laxatives

I've been through lots of different laxatives, and lots of different laxatives have been through me (sorry, couldn't resist). The products I have tried include senna pills (which do terrible things to my stomach and cause untold amounts of pain and cramping), milk of magnesia (more gentle than senna and fairly effective, tastes like chalk), weird chemical laxatives that contain things I can't even pronounce, glycerin suppositories, Lactulose (tastes like syrup, made me nauseous) and Epsom salts (taste really, really disgusting, especially mixed with orange juice).

Laxatives do work, and some really, really work, but they have two main flaws. First, they often cause additional pain, especially the strong ones that contain senna or harsh chemicals, and that pain can be very intense indeed. It's sometimes described as "griping" pain, which means "sharp, spasmodic pains in the bowel," which sounds about right. I once woke up on Christmas Day with some very festive cramps and had to camp out in the bathroom at 8 a.m. because of some senna pills. So you just trade one pain for another.

The second problem is that laxatives aren't a long-term solution. A common feature of an IBS gut is that it can swing from constipation to diarrhea and back again in the flush of a toilet, so if you use a laxative tonight you might get diarrhea tomorrow and be back to constipation by the next day. It's a fun little circle of distress, and patients can spend years trying to find that elusive balance between one extreme and the other.

Fiber supplements

I have used Normacol (sterculia fiber), Celevac tablets (methylcellulose), Citrucel powder (also methylcellulose), acacia fiber (known as Heather's Tummy Fiber), Lepicol (psyllium fiber, sold as Metamucil in the U.S.), Linusit Gold (linseed/flaxseed, not technically a fiber supplement, but it's often used in a similar way) and some really quite excruciatingly foul brown substance that called itself a colon cleanser and tasted more like horse dung than anything else.

I quite like fiber supplements. They do seem to help, and they can be taken every day with no worries as long as they contain no extra ingredients. They're certainly not a panacea, but I've taken them for a good few years now and I don't plan to stop anytime soon.

You can see how fiber supplements work if you put a big spoonful of fiber in a glass of water and leave it overnight. It swells up in a rather fun manner, and you can imagine it squidging down your colon and cleaning out everything in its path.

Some fibers seem to agree with me more than others. My guts hated the psyllium fiber, which caused more stomach pain than I'd had to begin with. The acacia fiber didn't seem to do much of anything, but I liked the Linusit Gold, which seemed to help for a while at least.

Normal and Celevac have definitely been the best fibers I've found. Normacol comes in little white grains that you swallow with water, which means it's very easy to take. Celevac comes in pink tablets that you chew, and it's harder to take as the tablets get stuck to your teeth, but it's not too bad. It becomes a rather boring daily routine, to sit and swallow this stuff and then drink a massive glass of water, but it's worth it.

Drugs

I have tried Colofac (an antispasmodic) and Buscopan (another antispasmodic). These drugs seem to have little or no effect on me, so I've never used them for very long.

It's unfortunate that the two breakthrough IBS drugs of recent times, Lotronex and Zelnorm, have never been approved for use in the U.K., despite the fact that they've been approved in countries like the U.S. for years. Many sufferers have benefited from these drugs, and it's tough to know that a possible treatment is available to millions of sufferers but not to you.

Having said that, at the time of writing, the use of Lotronex has been restricted in the U.S.A., and Zelnorm has been withdrawn completely, everywhere, because of safety concerns, so that's not much use to anyone. But it would have been nice to at least have had some kind of access to these modern drugs and to believe that if any more drugs get released in the future we Brits have a chance of getting hold of them.

It's a very strange situation if you think about it. How can a drug possibly be safe enough for American sufferers, but not for British ones? It can't, of course, and it's a situation created solely by the stringency of regulatory bodies in different countries, bodies that often seem to think that any risks from these drugs negate their genuine benefits because IBS is not life-threatening or "serious."

If you consider that I've had IBS for two decades and I've taken a grand total of two medications you can appreciate the plight of the IBS sufferer and the hapless doctors who try to treat us. There simply haven't been enough drugs developed for IBS. U.K. patients with diarrhea-predominant IBS take the same Imodium and Lomotil pills that they used thirty years ago, and patients with constipation take the same laxatives and stool softeners. American sufferers are given two brand-new drugs and then asked to give them up because a tiny number of people experienced side effects.

IBS is just not taken seriously by the medical profession or by drug companies. We deserve a miracle drug. Where's our Viagra?

Change in diet

The main dietary regimen I have used, and the one that has helped me the most, is a gluten-free diet. Although the absence of gluten really seems to agree with my bowel, it can be difficult to maintain. Whoever makes food these days really has it in for me, putting gluten in crisps, sausages, ready meals, soup . . . you name it, they put gluten in it.

Just about the only completely safe foods, the ones you can eat without reading the label, are the ones that don't actually *have* a label: fresh fruit and veggies, for example. I've been halfway through a slice of ham when I've thought, *Better just check the label,* and found "wheat starch" printed on it.

I am careful to avoid gluten, but not overly so. I eat sauces that contain gluten, for instance, because the amount of gluten in a sauce is so minimal it doesn't seem to make much difference. To avoid gluten 100 percent of the time would mean cooking absolutely everything from scratch, and I don't have the patience or the incentive for that, as I seem to be okay with a small amount of the stuff.

My overall diet is fairly healthy and I try to stick to as many non-processed foods as I can because it's common sense that my bowel will be less easily offended by chicken and veggies than by chicken and veggies plus 101 additives.

I have cut out tea, coffee and alcohol, as these drinks can affect even healthy guts. Instead of tea or coffee I drink red bush herbal tea and pure fruit juices, and I drink Coke if I'm in a pub or restaurant. I also drink a lot of water to make sure that all the fiber I take has a decent amount of liquid to combine with—usually a liter a day, half with my morning fiber dose and half with the evening dose.

There's absolutely no doubt that diet can affect IBS symptoms, but it's no more of an easy cure than any other treatment. It amazes me when people say their doctors have told them to simply "change" their diets, or, my personal favorite, "watch what you eat." What on earth are we supposed to be watching for? A label on the butter that says, "This stuff will mess your bowels up"? We're never told.

Occasionally a doctor will mention that we should identify our "trigger" foods and then avoid them, but this is no piece of cake either. Trigger foods (foods that trigger our symptoms) can take hours or even days to manifest themselves as pain. My symptoms tend to show up a full two or three days after I have eaten gluten, and that makes correlations between symptoms and food intake very tough to spot. For some diarrhea sufferers, the simple act of eating can be enough to trigger symptoms, regardless of what food you might be eating, so that complicates matters further.

Sufferers can also spend a lot of time looking for one or two individual foods to cut from their diets. For example, they'll decide that they're affected by oranges, whereas in reality a whole group of foods might be affecting them, or anything with citrus fruit buried in its ingredients. Examining your diet is an obvious step to take for IBS sufferers, but not an easy one.

One thing that we can all do is make sure that we're eating a basically healthy diet to begin with, one that makes it as easy for our guts as is humanly possible. I don't have much sympathy for people who drink ten cups of coffee a day and eat bacon for breakfast and McDonald's for lunch and then complain about their bowel habits—that's not IBS, that's normal biology. Our digestive system was not designed to run on junk, and everyone knows that what goes in affects what comes out. You can't expect to eat half your weight in water buffalo and not get sick, and someone who is eating a diet that consists of sugar, fat and all things garbage can't complain about their guts; their guts should complain about them.

Hypnotherapy

My face-to-face hypnotherapy sessions were nice and relaxing, if not hugely helpful. The hypnotherapist was a very kind man who treated me with respect and listened to me carefully rather than making assumptions and judging me, and that was soothing in itself.

Hypnotherapy wasn't a cure for me by any means, but it was still rather enjoyable. There's no doubt that hypnotherapy is one of the most respected treatments for IBS, and there are plenty of clinical trials to show that it's effective and plenty of doctors who recommend it. It seems a no-brainer to me to try this particular therapy, as it is tried and tested and comes with the promise of no side effects whatsoever.

I also tried the IBS Audio Program 100, which unfortunately didn't seem to do much for me, although again it was certainly calming and relaxing.

Over-the-counter supplements

The OTC supplements I have tried include peppermint pills, magnesium supplements, vitamin C, friendly bacteria supplements such as acidophilus and other probiotics, and aloe vera juice.

The peppermint pills (Colpermin) really didn't do much. They were the enteric-coated kind, which means that they are designed to dissolve only when they reach the intestine instead of dissolving in the stomach. Apparently for some people they calm the guts down and even make your gas smell delightful (and who wouldn't want that), but they didn't do that for me.

The magnesium pills definitely helped, and I still take these in the form of magnesium citrate. For constipation sufferers magnesium can have a laxative effect (think of milk of magnesia), and calcium is the equivalent remedy for diarrhea sufferers. Calcium carbonate is probably the type of calcium used most often for diarrhea, sometimes with vitamin D included in the pills as well. Caltrate Plus is a famous calcium brand in the U.S.A.

Vitamin C apparently has a laxative effect at high doses, and I once tried a powder form of it that tasted like radioactive sherbet. It was quite fun to take, but it didn't help my bowels.

Friendly bacteria in the form of probiotics are great in theory, but not for me in practice. I've tried them in pills, drinks and a special super-concentrated powder that was supposed to have seven gajillion bugs in it and even that didn't help. Aloe vera made me go to the bathroom but also gave me intestinal spasms, so that was no good either.

I'm not sure if this final item should go in the supplement section or the diet section, but I once tried eating a load of raw garlic because it was supposed to kill bad bacteria or candida or some other such thing. I don't think it killed any bad bacteria but it undoubtedly almost killed me.

Homeopathic remedy

To be honest, I'm slightly ashamed to admit that I've tried homeopathy. I have no problem with some complementary therapies such as acupuncture, because at least if you're sticking needles into someone there's a genuine chance that you might be physically changing something within their body, but homeopathy seems completely far-fetched.

It basically relies on the idea that the more diluted the treatment, the more potent it is, so the best homeopathic treatments are so diluted they are almost completely comprised of water. The best argument I have heard against homeopathy is the question of what happens when the homeopaths wash their beakers out. Don't they end up with a solution so potent it could blow up the world?

The fact that I tried something I thought was ridiculous tells you how desperate I was for relief. The homeopathic treatment I tried was in pill form, and as far as I can remember it was a treatment designed for constipation. I think it may have been *nux vomica,* which Google tells me is indeed a remedy for constipated people as well as for people who are "disposed to reproach others" and have "dreams full of bustle and hurry."

I seem to remember getting a bit of a stomachache when I took the pills, but that could have been a coincidence rather than the effect of that one-in-a-million particle of whatever stuff was supposed to be in there.

Heating pad

One of my frustrations over the years has been that all of my symptoms are not only invisible but also inaccessible to any kind of hands-on, mechanical manipulation. At least when I was having back problems I could go to an osteopath and have my back squished to make it better, but there's no equivalent for IBS. Occasionally I would try to press on my stomach and massage it to release what felt like a buildup of air, and that would help for a few seconds, but then the bloated feeling would return.

The only "hands-on" thing that helps me is a heating pad. My pad is a mini version of an electric blanket; you just plug it in and put it on the bit of you that hurts. I use it for the really brutal pain attacks (when I'm not sitting on the toilet). While it doesn't take the pain away entirely, it does take the edge off a little.

* * *

And that's it. I have to admit that I've never taken perhaps the most famous IBS friend of all—Imodium. I haven't ever tried Imodium because I tend to get more constipation than diarrhea, and when I do have a diarrhea flareup it lasts for only a few hours or an afternoon. I worry that taking Imodium would just be booking myself in for more constipation to come.

I feel like a bit of a fraud here. What kind of paid-up member of the IBS classes has not even tried our flagship drug? But I hope I've proved my IBS credentials without needing to take Imodium. Maybe one day I'll try it, just for fun.

CHAPTER 17

Top Tips for IBS Sufferers

LET'S END THIS LONG IBS TALE WITH SOME TIPS that might come in useful if your own IBS symptoms are ruling and ruining your life. I wish I could tell you that you just need to follow a gluten-free diet and use the same supplements that I do to find relief, but the reality is that IBS has many different manifestations and each sufferer needs to find an individual special remedy.

However, I do think there are a number of things that any IBS sufferer can do in the quest for health and a better quality of life. The last thing I want is for you to finish this book and end up twice as miserable as when you started (assuming you were miserable when you started; you may have been as happy as a clam, I don't know). While my story has been a painful one, it does have a decent happy ending. You deserve that, too.

So if you haven't found your route to better health yet, here are some ideas that you might like to try, culled from my two decades of IBS experience.

Keep up the reading

The more you know about IBS, the better. When I started investigating the treatments available to me, I was amazed to find a whole range of pills, potions and therapies that I had no idea existed. If you haven't even heard of hypnotherapy, magnesium, calcium, fiber supplements, peppermint pills or antispasmodics, you are never going to be in a position to try them.

A good general knowledge of IBS also helps me immensely when I start to feel sorry for myself. Simply knowing that it is one of the most common health problems in the country helps a great deal. I may feel like the only person in the world who cannot control her own bowels, but every time I go out, I probably see five other people with the same condition. I am completely normal and so are you.

You know your body better than anyone

If you have suffered from IBS for any length of time, you have become an expert on your own symptoms. Your doctor might recommend eating more bran (some doctors still haven't read the studies that prove bran equals pain for many IBS patients) when you know categorically that bran makes you ill. It's important that you trust your expertise. If you know that a particular food or situation always gives you pain, then it doesn't matter what anyone else says—you're the only person who has lived within your body and you know best.

Keep records

I could have saved myself a lot of time and effort if I had kept careful records of exactly what supplements I was taking during my so-called mystery year of wellness. Instead, I had to rack my brain to try to remember the exact brands and dosages and even then it took some experimenting before I got things right.

It has to be said that keeping a record of every last thing you swallow is very dull indeed, and it can often seem fruitless because you can't see any correlation between the things you are ingesting and your health. However, I would suggest that there are two situations where it can be truly useful to keep detailed records: when you are feeling very ill and when you are feeling great. If you are careful to record the circumstances that lead to these two extremes, you might spot something that is triggering your attacks in the bad times or staving off the symptoms in the good times.

Try not to be embarrassed

This is a difficult one. There are many facets of IBS which can be mortifying, and if you've just been incontinent in front of sundry friends and relatives then it takes real courage to hold your head up high and face the world. But I would encourage you to try and to not let the symptoms grind you down.

After many years of being embarrassed I can now talk about IBS pretty easily with my family and friends. It has almost become routine for me to refer to my condition in everyday conversation. That doesn't mean that I bring up intimate details of my toilet habits over afternoon tea, but it does mean that I'm never scared of talking about my condition.

If we try not to be embarrassed, we're not only making things better for ourselves, we're also making things better for all the other sufferers who follow us. Every time you talk about IBS openly it enables someone else to do the same, and if they're talking about the problem they're on the way to finding help. If you take a matter-of-fact attitude toward bodily functions, you'll probably find that the people around you will take your cue. And if anyone laughs, then they're a cretin and you can tell them I said so.

Having said all that, you are also entitled to keep quiet about your IBS if you want to. I wouldn't recommend trying to keep it a secret from close family and friends, but to anyone else your private medical concerns are just that, private.

There's nothing wrong with saying you have a vague digestive problem or a food allergy or whatever else you feel comfortable with if you don't want to say you have an irritable bowel, and if people try to stick their noses into your business you should tell them to butt out.

Find other sufferers and have a good moan

The irony of IBS is that you often feel very alone, despite the fact that it's so common. Western societies consider it taboo to talk about toilet functions and we teach our children that poop is disgusting and not to be mentioned. This attitude often continues into adulthood—how many people do you know who come into work and say, "Well *that* crap was more trouble than it was worth"?

It is vital, though, that we let ourselves talk about these things or we will never find the help that we deserve. I have heard from embarrassed sufferers who have waited years and years before going to the doctor, suffering all the while. It's terrible that people are so ashamed of their problems they feel like they can't ask for help.

There is support available, and the Internet in particular is a wonderful way for people with bowel problems to talk about their symptoms openly. Take a look at www.ibstales.com for hundreds of personal stories from IBS sufferers just like you.

Don't give up!

IBS can be overwhelming. It can feel like your troubles are never-ending and you will never be able to live a normal life. But please don't stop looking for solutions. If your doctor says he can do nothing for you then find another doctor. Ask for a referral to a gastroenterologist, and if he just sticks his finger up your rectum try another one.

Have a read through the stories on IBS Tales and see if you can find a fiber supplement or medication or alternative therapy that might help. If your friends aren't sympathetic then show them this book, or write your own IBS story down, send it to www.ibstales.com and give your friends the web address. Let them read about your suffering and the suffering of hundreds of others and dare them to laugh.

Many people find that it takes them a while to find the right treatment for their symptoms, but they do find it, in a diet or a supplement or a therapy. Maybe you'll be helped by one of the new drugs being developed for IBS; your relief might be right round the corner.

There is always hope, no matter how bad things get. Never forget that many thousands of IBS sufferers have found ways to tame the dreaded beast of the bowel and live normal, healthy lives. There's an answer out there for you too.

How to contact me

If you have any questions or comments about this book I would love to hear from you! Just visit www.ibstales.com and contact me through the site.

I wish you the very best of luck in your battle with IBS. May you find the support, understanding and relief that you deserve. Be strong and stand up for yourself. And if you don't have the strength to do that at the moment, come and visit my website and we can all stand up together.

About the Author

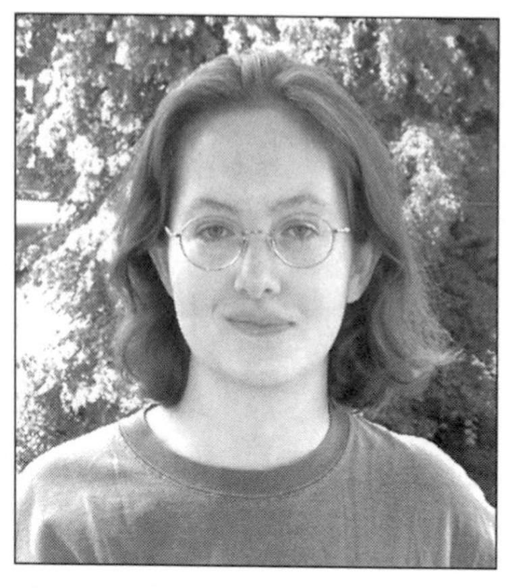

Sophie Lee has suffered from irritable bowel syndrome since she was 12 years old. Symptoms of diarrhea, constipation, pain and bloating dominated her life for almost twenty years until she finally found a way to control her symptoms and get her life back.

She runs the IBS Tales website at www.ibstales.com where hundreds of IBS sufferers meet to tell the truth about what it really means to live with IBS.

Sophie has a degree in English literature and a postgraduate diploma in journalism. She was born and brought up in the United Kingdom and lives on the south coast of England.